The ANTI-DIET

Workbook

break the diet cycle,
practice intuitive eating,
and **live** with total food freedom

Brandy Minks
MS, RDN, CD, CNSC

ULYSSES PRESS

Published by:
ULYSSES PRESS
PO Box 3440
Berkeley, CA 94703
www.ulyssespress.com

ISBN: 978-1-64604-309-5
Library of Congress Control Number: 2021946380

Printed in the United States by Kingery Printing Company
10 9 8 7 6 5 4 3 2 1

Acquisitions editor: Ashten Evans
Managing editor: Claire Chun
Editor: Kathy Kaiser
Proofreader: Renee Rutledge
Front cover design: Justin Shirley
Interior design: what!design @ whatweb.com
Production: Jake Flaherty

NOTE TO READERS: This book has been written and published strictly for informational purposes, and in no way should it be used as a substitute for consultation with your medical doctor or health-care professional. All facts in this book came from medical files, clinical journals, scientific publications, personal interviews, published trade books, self-published materials by experts, magazine articles, and the personal-practice experiences of the authorities quoted or sources cited. You should not consider educational material herein to be the practice of medicine or to replace consultation with a physician or other medical practitioner. The author and publisher are providing you with information in this work so that you can have the knowledge and can choose, at your own risk, to act on that knowledge. The author and publisher also urge all readers to be aware of their health status and to consult health professionals before beginning any health program, including changes in dietary habits.

To whom I've harmed with diets:
I'm sorry, and I hope you can find food freedom.

Contents

Introduction

Dear Reader,

I'm so excited that you have picked up this book! It means you are interested in changing your outlook on your body and how you view health. There is a movement in the world today called Health at Every Size (HAES), which promotes body acceptance and sheds light on our society's bias against higher-weight bodies. Along with this movement is the intuitive eating (IE) framework, famous for leading people out of the dieting and weight loss world, and into a healthier relationship with food and the body. I will be referring to both HAES and IE, but in addition to this workbook, I encourage you to read books devoted to these topics (see appendix A for recommended titles and more).

There are a few things I need to mention before you delve in. I am an "anti-diet" dietitian. I do not condone dieting for weight loss or using weight loss as a treatment for illness. In treating my patients, I do not provide food or calorie restriction. As you'll read in this book, there are many diets or restrictive eating patterns that can cause harm. Being anti-diet does not mean that I disregard well-researched medical nutrition therapy to treat specific diseases, such as for kidney disease. If you are following a certain diet to treat a condition, this does not mean that you can't do intuitive eating! If you do have a special diet, I highly recommend working with a certified IE dietitian, who can provide specific guidance for your body's needs.

In this book I use weight and calorie numbers in certain chapters as they pertain to my own story, to the stories of my patients (whose names I have changed to protect their identities), and to body mass index (BMI) and other research presented. Other anti-diet books tend to remove these numbers, as they can sometimes trigger negative feelings in the reader or even become a how-to guide for someone looking for the next diet to try. I use numbers in certain parts of this book where I need them to prove my points. Stay aware of your feelings as you read and skip over parts as you need to.

THE **ANTI-DIET** WORKBOOK

Now let's talk about verbiage. I use the word "fat" in this book in a literal sense. While the term is considered derogatory slang, fat people are reclaiming it as a descriptor, just like calling someone tall. The same approach has been used in the LGTBQ+ community, where they embrace terms that have historically been used to shame and marginalize them. Terms such as "obese" or "overweight" are considered weight-stigmatizing as they pathologize higher-weight bodies. I use these "O" words on occasion in this text when talking about pertinent research (such as in Chapter 2), but I mostly use neutral descriptive words.

This workbook is intended for the person who is ready to develop a better relationship with their body and rediscover the intuitive eater we all have within. You may be unhappy with your body. You may have attempted diets in order to lose weight, change your body size, or get healthier. Or you may have disordered eating habits or a disordered mindset around food or your body. The following are descriptions of some disordered eating practices as well as common eating disorders. A person may have disordered eating if they exhibit any of these behaviors in part or in whole (in Chapter 4, you will take a quiz to help you determine what specific disordered eating behaviors you may exhibit). People with disordered eating are at higher risk for developing an eating disorder.

- **Binge eating:** This behavior results from restriction (physical restriction, such as eating fewer calories or avoiding certain foods, or mental restriction, such as telling yourself you will stop bingeing starting tomorrow), which leads to strong food cravings. Bingeing is associated with eating an unusually large amount of food in one sitting; the person who binges feels guilt and shame for having eaten so much and typically feels out of control with food.

- **Orthorexia:** The person with this condition spends an abnormal amount of time thinking about food and health. They are obsessed with eating only the "right" foods or what they deem the "healthiest" foods. They may have food rules that do not allow them to eat "unhealthy" foods, or they may eliminate certain foods from their diet in pursuit of health. Other behaviors typical for this person are tracking calories or macronutrients; compulsively checking food labels and ingredient lists; writing down everything they eat; showing high levels of distress or anxiety when "healthy" foods are not available; and constantly thinking about the next meal.

- **Emotional eating:** The person who eats this way does so to soothe their emotional state, not because they are physically hungry. They might eat when faced with any emotion, but will typically do so when negative feelings arise, such as sadness, anger, anxiety, stress, depression, fear, loneliness, or even boredom (we'll talk about emotional eating in more depth in Chapter 4 when we discuss intuitive eating). Emotional eating is not always disordered but can be if it leads to further distress or bingeing.

- **Eating in secret:** The person who eats in secret waits to eat until they are alone and does not want others to see or judge them for the type or amount of food they are eating. This could look like accepting a treat from a coworker but waiting until they are alone in the car to eat it; waking up in the night to have a snack so that others living with them do not see; or hiding food wrappers so that no one sees the wrappers in the trash.

- **Bulimia nervosa:** The person with bulimia nervosa eats a large amount of food in a short period of time and then induces purging through vomiting, laxatives, or other methods. This person often feels shame and guilt about their eating and may have body dysmorphia.

- **Anorexia nervosa:** The person with this condition severely restricts calories or exercises excessively to expend calories to lose weight or prevent weight gain. This person has an extreme fear of gaining weight or having a larger body size and may have body dysmorphia.

All of these disordered eating practices and eating disorders usually come with a side of poor body image. Here are some other examples of disordered mindset around food and body:

- The person perceives that they are bigger in size than they actually are.

- The person is fearful of gaining weight.

- The person is anxious about attending social events, fearing a loss of control around food.

- The person feels undeserving of romance, friendship, a career, new clothing, happiness, and so on, until they reach their desired weight.

- The person thinks in terms of "all or nothing." They are fully committed to a diet in the beginning, but when motivation fails and they "cheat," the diet is over. This person feels guilty that they failed. This often leads to binge eating right before and after restricting their food.

- The person has poor self-confidence because of body size. The person often displays the qualities of an introvert. They do not want to participate in group events for fear of being "seen" and therefore judged or bullied because of their weight or size. This person will likely not move out of their comfort zone with activities such as changing jobs, traveling, giving a speech at a wedding, going dancing, and so on.

Many people with the behaviors and mindsets just described may not realize that they have a problem. Often, disordered eating behaviors go unrecognized, as going on a diet or losing weight is considered healthy in our society. A 2008 study from the University of North Carolina at Chapel Hill showed that a shocking 65 percent of US women between the ages of 25 and 45 have disordered eating behaviors.[1] Diet culture is to blame.

What is diet culture? This is a complex topic, but briefly, diet culture is the perception that weight loss should be prioritized because fat is bad and thin is good, healthy, and beautiful. You have probably seen evidence of diet culture in the media, such as when celebrities are praised for weight loss and they share their dieting tips and tricks. Or you may have seen loved ones in your own life trying to diet to lose weight. It is likely that at some point someone has made a comment about your body or what you were eating. This could even have been a doctor or health care professional telling you that you needed to lose weight in the name of health. In Western society, skinny is seen as successful. All the seemingly "normal" dieting practices in society are actually quite harmful and can lead to the disordered habits and mindsets discussed.

In the next chapter, I will tell you about my own experience growing up in diet culture, why I decided to become a dietitian, and how I went from working in the weight loss industry to fighting for the Health at Every Size movement. Then I'll discuss the research that explains how dieting and weight loss attempts are harmful. I will show you the

---

1   "Survey Finds Disoriented Eating Behaviors Among Three Out of Four American Women (Fall, 2008)," *Carolina Public Health Magazine.*

research about intuitive eating and how you can reject diet culture. By the time you are ready to jump into the workbook, you'll have a good understanding of the intuitive eating framework and be ready to do some healing work.

The workbook is a set of guided journaling prompts and activities to help you practice intuitive eating and take steps toward body acceptance. Recovery from disordered eating and diet culture is not a linear path. There will be a lot of unlearning and relearning along the way. Because diet culture is not something we can readily escape, you will work on building your resilience, learning to trust your body and yourself again.

You will be using meditation and mindfulness to reconnect with your body and food. The journaling prompts and guided activities are to help you cultivate a mindset of gratefulness, body acceptance, and self-awareness. Now is a time to rekindle self-love, self-compassion, empathy, confidence, and happiness.

So with that, jump into the first chapter!

Warmly,

Brandy

Chapter 1

My Story

I grew up in a thin, tall body and had thin, tall parents and thin siblings. No one in my household actively dieted, but my mom tried to emphasize eating "healthy." We rarely ate out or had sugary cereals in the house, but I think the main reason was because money was tight. We ate meals together at the kitchen table. Like many kids, I remember not being allowed dessert until I ate a certain amount of dinner (I could never finish those lima beans—yuck!).

Sweets were my love. Seven- or eight-year-old me would sneak into the kitchen after everyone had gone to bed to find the candy on top of the fridge. I would enlist my sisters to distract my mom during the day so I could pillage the candy in her workroom. Halloween or Christmas candy was gone in a matter of days. And my favorite store was the "candy store," a corner store just up the street, where my dad would take my siblings and me once a week. When I had money, I would beg my parents to let me walk up to that store to buy treats. They usually said yes, but I will never forget the disappointed looks from my mom.

I was about ten when I saw a huge, fuzzy Valentine's Day teddy bear in a drugstore. The bear was too expensive for my mom to justify buying. But she thought she would teach me a lesson in saving my money and paid me to help her wind shuttles for her weaving work. I had saved up $20 by the time we went back. Unfortunately, the bear was gone. But my disappointment lasted only thirty seconds. Then I came up with plan B: I would spend my money on treats! I gathered up all kinds of candy, soda, and chips. My mom kept trying to change my mind, showing me other toys and encouraging me to save the money for something that would last longer. But nothing could change my determined mind. I had a grand tea party that afternoon with all my snacks.

At age eleven, I started to become aware of how people were talking about bodies. Family events were often filled with diet talk. Many of my extended family members were fat and had tried numerous diets over the years. I overheard lots of conversations about the diets they were on and saw them drinking lots of light beer. At school I noticed that bigger kids were teased about their size. Being fat was decidedly a bad thing.

As I started middle school, I became more aware of my own body. I was teased for wearing "high-water" jeans, which were too short in the leg and showed my ankles. I was already taller than most kids in my grade, and finding pants that fit were often an issue. People would comment on my skinny body, often calling me "beanpole." They didn't mean it in a bad way though. It almost felt like a compliment, and it reinforced my belief that my body size was desirable. Around seventh or eighth grade, I started watching what I was eating when I was away from home. In the school lunch line, I would grab the optional vegetable of the day, typically carrots, and eat them sans dressing. Although I craved the cookies and Rice Krispies Treats, I rarely allowed myself to buy them because I wanted everyone to see that I was eating healthy. When I got home from school, the kitchen was my first stop. If there wasn't anything sweet readily available, I would create something myself, thus beginning my love for cooking and baking. My go-to option was a cereal snack consisting of marshmallows, peanut butter, and chocolate chips melted down and combined with whatever cereal was around, such as Kix or Cheerios. Or I would utilize my Easy-Bake Oven and boxed cake mix (usually eating lots of batter because I was not able to wait until the light bulb cooked it!).

I had a few trusted friends that I would enjoy candy or treats in front of, but I noticed they never seemed to have a desire for sugar like I did. Candy or other treats could last for weeks or months in their houses versus a day or two in mine. I found myself drifting back to their kitchens when no one was looking to find another treat. One time I even ate half a bottle of gummy multivitamins and was very embarrassed when my friend's mom noticed.

As I started high school, my desire to eat healthier got stronger. I dreamed of having a flat stomach like many of the actresses or singers I loved. My first semester I took a nutrition class that ended up being more of a cooking class. I'm extremely thankful that there wasn't a huge emphasis on calorie counting or classifying foods as good or bad (I did enough of that on my own). I think my own lack of knowledge about these things may have prevented more seriously disordered eating habits. I really liked cooking and baking, and I started doing more of this at home. I collected cookbooks and recipes. My parents even bought me an apron and recipe binder with blank pages to write out recipes. I still have that binder. It has recipes from that nutrition class and from a few Pillsbury holiday recipe books, but mostly it is filled with dessert recipes that I hand copied out of books or magazines, along with pictures of some of those desserts, cut out from the magazines and pasted into the binder.

Around this time, I started checking out old issues of *Self* and other health magazines from the library. I would do the exercises from the magazines in my room, mainly the abdominal exercises. I eventually got my own yearly subscription to a few of these magazines and would cut out the pages with recipes and exercises to tape to my bedroom wall. I continued to eat more nutritiously at school and sugar binge when I got home. My junior year of high school I joined the dance team, thinking that maybe I just needed to exercise more to compensate for my eating habits. Maybe then I would have visible abs.

That same year, my grandma Marilyn and I started taking cooking classes at a natural grocery store as a way to spend more one-on-one time together. I learned the art of making pies, I learned how to cook fish, and I learned that I loved piroshki. Being in a natural foods market, the instructors always had something to say about the ingredients: which ones were more sustainable or why organic was best. I loved learning about different cuisines and flavor combinations. I thought maybe my future career would be something culinary. But lo and behold, my favorite class was one taught by a retired dietitian. I don't even remember what foods we made, but I remember her sharing her food science knowledge and being inspired. She taught us what kinds of ingredients were more nutritious than others and the effects they had in preventing or treating disease. My orthorexia brain perked up and I suddenly knew what I was going to study at college: nutrition!

My freshman year at Washington State University challenged my ability to hide my sugar binges. I shared a dorm room with my soon-to-be best friend, so I didn't have much time alone. I also was adjusting to obtaining most of my food from the huge cafeterias. There was now an even bigger audience of people who could see what was on my tray—and I was going to be a dietitian. Strangers couldn't see me eating something unhealthy, so I never once partook of the ice cream or slushy machines, the dessert bar, or the soda fountain. I stuck to the salad bar and the wrap station, and occasionally I got a burger from the grill.

I was very active that year. I walked all over campus for classes, went on exploration walks or runs with my roommate, and walked to the gym for more cardio and ab workouts a few times a week. As a result, my cravings for sugar were through the roof. Because all the student stores and little markets were run by my peers, I rarely felt comfortable buying the candy I wanted. I tried making the switch to dried fruit or chocolate protein bars. I would get yogurt and put it in the freezer to pretend it was ice cream. One day I finally worked up the nerve to buy what I really wanted: a jar of Nutella. The spoon went into the peanut butter jar and then the Nutella jar—no time for bread. I don't remember how long that Nutella was around, but I remember trying to make it last at least a week so my roommate wouldn't think I was crazy.

At social events, I would eat what everyone else ate and enjoy a small dessert to seem like I was fitting in. I even had friends comment that they liked seeing a nutrition major eat cookies. Maybe it gave them some peace about their own eating habits. I loved food and enjoyed opportunities to join a group for frozen yogurt or go out to eat. When I was in a group of friends, I felt that my food choices wouldn't be scrutinized as closely.

After I was accepted into the rigorous dietetic program, I moved to Spokane, Washington, for my classes. I felt pressure to be even more on top of my health game. I was training to be an expert. I couldn't let my classmates or other health-focused students on campus see me bring pizza for lunch. All the social groups I fell in with also had a desire to eat healthy and would ask me for my opinion on coconut oil or if I thought dairy was okay to eat. I didn't have a regular escape from health talk until my fiancé left the Air Force and got an apartment near mine. I finally felt I had a place to go where I didn't have to hide the fact that I wanted Taco Bell or to eat candy or snacks all evening.

Once we were married, we lived in an apartment complex that was within walking distance of major grocery stores and fast-food chains. Almost daily, we would walk down to Safeway for dinner and treats. After we had made our selections, I typically waited outside the store for him to go through the checkout. I was anxious that someone I knew would see me buying the "junk" food and think I wasn't a good dietetic student.

I was still embarrassed that I couldn't control myself when I got cravings—although it wasn't for lack of trying. In my classes I learned how to help someone track their food and calorie intake for weight loss and tried implementing it myself. I thought if I could just lose 10 pounds I would have the perfect body (even though I was already fairly thin). My efforts didn't last long. I found tracking my calories tedious, and I didn't believe what I tracked was accurate. Even though I wasn't really hungry, I couldn't break my habit of snacking in the evenings. An educated guess would be that my stress levels from school and work contributed to this.

My dual program in Nutrition and Exercise Physiology was extremely demanding. There were many days and weeks when I was barely holding it together. On top of my nutrition and counseling classes, I also had exercise physiology, electrocardiogram, and exercise prescription classes. Of course, the central focus of all the nutrition and exercise-based treatments I was learning was weight loss. From diabetes to arthritis to cancer, a higher BMI was always taught to be a risk factor. Nutrition counseling centered on helping a person lose weight in order to prevent or improve disease, and little was taught on just treating the disease itself. My teachers made it seem as though only fat people had diseases.

In my senior year, we ran a free clinic that was open to the public. It was to give us experience practicing the counseling skills we were taught in the classroom. I remember feeling inadequate when it came to helping my clients. We had only basic textbook knowledge at this point, no medical nutrition therapy classes or shadowing of dietitians in the field. I was assigned a very nice woman who had been coming to the free clinic for a few years. She wanted to lose weight and thought if she had weekly check-ins, it would motivate her and hold her more accountable. She would always attempt the things I suggested: calorie restriction, write down everything she ate, exercise three times a week, drink lots of water, and so on. But usually she would fall back into her old habits of hitting the drive-through on the way home from work and eating whatever she wanted on the weekends. I was at a loss for how to help her other than to be a motivational speaker for her once a week. I felt her struggle because I couldn't control my own eating, but there was no way I would admit that.

At some point, one of my fellow dietetic students introduced me to intuitive eating. Our professor even let her give a presentation to the class on the subject. I remember really liking the idea of it, but not connecting how to apply it in the work we were doing. It wasn't obvious how it would work with diets we were learning about, such as a diabetic or DASH (Dietary Approaches to Stop Hypertension) diet. I think I believed it was only for people who had eating disorders, which at the time I had no training in. I also didn't think that intuitive eating could apply to me. Intuitive eating was pushed to the back of my mind to make room for knowledge that was going to actually be on my exams.

During my master's program and internship, there were many times I recommended weight loss interventions to patients. Many people in the diabetes clinic or Women, Infants, and Children (WIC) program were asking for meal plans or exercise routines that would promote weight loss. There was one patient during my hospital rotation, however, whom I really did not want to go talk to. This woman could have been on the show *My 600-lb Life*. Doctors and nurses pressured the dietitian and me to speak with her about her weight. I remember going to talk to her and feeling her tension start to build as soon as I told her who I was. She immediately started crying while trying to explain her size and what she was doing to try to lose weight. I listened patiently and didn't offer any advice. She was obviously distressed and overwhelmed with the amount of weight loss talk she'd been receiving. I truly felt bad for her, and at the same time couldn't wrap my brain around how someone could possibly let themselves get that large.

Fast-forward to my first job: a dietitian in a weight loss clinic. The clinic had a medical weight loss program and a bariatric surgery program (not uncommon for most weight loss clinics). In the beginning, the clinic was small. The provider team was made up of two doctors, two surgeons, and three dietitians, including myself. Over six months we expanded our clinical team quickly as the patient wait list grew. I was trained in both programs and felt I was making a difference. My superiors gave me very specific training in the art of inducing weight loss. After struggling to help people lose weight during my college years, I finally felt I had the secret weapon to actually help my patients control their weight and improve their health.

Many of the patients had similar life goals that they thought would be achieved through weight loss. They wanted to get off all medications; better control their chronic disease(s); stop family and doctors from pestering them about their weight; feel better about themselves; not be out of breath when climbing a hill or stairs; fit comfortably in an airplane or roller coaster seat; have more energy; live longer; prevent disability; and so on. All of these were valid goals and I too thought weight loss alone would be the solution for them.

In the medical weight loss program, I assessed my patients holistically: I reviewed their diet, hydration status, exercise routine, stress levels, gut health, sleep habits, lab values, diagnoses, and medications. I taught my patients the Mediterranean diet, portion control, meal planning, how to write grocery lists, and stress management. I provided recipes, set up calorie restriction, promoted eating every two to three hours, and developed exercise plans. When the patient insisted, I sometimes facilitated other diets, such as the ketogenic diet or the elimination diet.

For a whole year I thought I was killing it. I was teaching my patients everything they needed to know to lose weight and be healthy. Almost all my patients had dieted before and actually had a lot of nutrition knowledge. I thought maybe these people just needed an extra push once a month from the doctor or myself to keep them going. I found most patients had moderate success at first, meaning they lost 0.5 to 2 pounds per week, maybe around 10 to 20 pounds total (that is, before they gained it back a year or two later). Only a handful of patients had a big weight loss achievement, such as losing 50 to 100 pounds, through diet alone. I assumed they were super successful because they were highly motivated and making all the "right" lifestyle changes.

But those who struggled to lose weight and keep it off puzzled me. In this situation, my mentors would recommend I restrict calories further, put the patient on weight loss shakes and bars for a few weeks, or talk with the doctor about adding a medication, such as an appetite suppressant, to help move things along. They even suggested that the patient might be lying about making lifestyle changes. I didn't think my patients were lying. It seemed like a big mystery. Why could some patients lose weight while others could not? Why would some regain weight in a short time even without reverting to their old habits?

One patient's story has stuck with me. Mandy was a woman in her thirties who came to the weight loss clinic worried about her health. She said she wasn't unhappy with her body but had been told by all her health care providers that she was in danger of major disease and a short life if she did not lose weight. She did not have any outright medical problems at the time. She hadn't dieted before and wasn't sure where to start. She knew she did not want bariatric surgery, but she wanted to lose 100 pounds or more. Mandy's weight loss was extremely slow. She would plateau after a few weeks on her meal plan, and then I would readjust her calories and she could lose a little more. In our whole time working together, she only had small weight loss successes and then no weight loss for many months. Frustrated, she attempted all the different weight loss medication options and even tried keto for a short time (she saw that her brother had lost weight this way), and she still had minimal weight loss and sometimes weight regain. I thought about her often outside of work, wondering what else she could try to jump-start weight loss again. Mandy was getting so frustrated that she was starting to consider surgery. I noticed her attitude around her body had changed. She was mad at her body for the weight refusing to budge and would openly criticize herself.

This was one thing that always caught me off guard. Many of my patients would talk negatively about themselves. Comments such as "I hate this spare tire around my middle" or "I'm so fat and ugly" were common in my office. They were their own worst bully. I didn't know what to say when they would voice these complaints. I was scared to say the wrong thing and make them feel worse. I had never heard so many people talk about themselves in this way. Almost everyone had something negative to say. Most were mad at their bodies and themselves for never being able to lose weight and keep it off. I knew it was a problem.

As time went on, some practices that were the norm in our clinic started to seem strange. For example, many of my patients were prescribed medication by the doctor to assist in weight loss. As a dietitian, I felt medications for weight loss were a fad diet thing to do. I had grown up with the idea that medications were chemicals and that natural was better. Plus, these meds did not always help the patient develop healthy habits. Sometimes a person would come to the clinic only because they knew they could be prescribed diet pills. But it was a normal occurrence, and I eventually found myself discussing them as an option with my struggling patients. It wasn't until after I left my job at the weight loss clinic and talked to other doctors that I realized many of the medications prescribed for weight loss were troublesome.

Phentermine was a popular option. It's an appetite suppressant that also improves concentration and is sometimes prescribed off-label for people with attention deficit hyperactivity disorder (ADHD). This was typically the first drug discussed. Before starting phentermine, patients would have blood work done to see if they had good kidney function, and they would also have an electrocardiogram (ECG) done to ensure there was no heart issue.

I learned later that this drug was not being prescribed as intended by its creator. The doctors were prescribing it for long-term use, even going so far as to tell patients they might have to be on phentermine for life if they didn't want their appetite to come roaring back. But phentermine is not intended for long-term use.[2] There is a risk of addiction, there are potential cardiac side effects, and there are worrisome medication interactions (and typically my patients were on many medications). When a patient would become "tolerant" of their phentermine dose (meaning it was no longer doing the trick), the doctor would usually increase the dose instead of discontinuing it as the manufacturer suggests. Those poor patients were guinea pigs, as there was little randomized control trial research published at the time showing the safety of long-term phentermine use.

Another drug often prescribed for weight loss was Wellbutrin, an antidepressant that sometimes has the side effect of appetite suppression. That's right, I said "sometimes." Wellbutrin seemed to be hit or miss in promoting weight loss. Patients with depression sometimes did benefit mentally from this prescription, but too often I saw it prescribed for patients without a diagnosis or symptoms of depression. I remember a pharmaceutical company representative came to the office once to promote Contrave, a mix of naltrexone, which is typically prescribed for alcohol and opioid dependence, and Wellbutrin. Approved by the FDA for weight loss management in 2014, Contrave was

---

2   "Phentermine," *LiverTox: Clinical and Research Information on Drug-Induced Liver Injury* (Bethesda, MD: National Institute of Diabetes and Digestive and Kidney Diseases, 2020). www.ncbi.nlm.nih.gov/books/NBK547916.

touted as a drug that could reduce food cravings and depress appetite. But such promises came with unnerving side effects: nausea, constipation, seizure, changes in mood or behavior, and even manic episodes.[3] It was unclear to me if these drugs really worked or maybe just had a placebo effect. In any case, there isn't much research to support their effectiveness in promoting long-term weight loss.

Metformin, an oral drug typically reserved for diabetics or prediabetics, was also prescribed to jump-start weight loss. This medication has many effects on the body but is known for decreasing blood sugar and improving insulin resistance, which is thought to cause weight gain. In our clinic, Metformin was prescribed even in patients without diabetes who were having trouble losing weight with diet and exercise alone. Research has shown that taking Metformin can lead to some gradual weight loss but mainly in patients who already have some degree of insulin resistance.[4] Side effects are often gastrointestinal distress, such as diarrhea, stomach cramps, or bloating. Although Metformin seems to be the least likely to cause serious harm of all the drugs mentioned, these patients were likely wasting their money and hopes on Metformin, especially if their blood work did not indicate they had insulin resistance.

An area I grew to really dislike was the bariatric surgery program. I felt like I was dangling a carrot in front of these patients. They did whatever we instructed them to do to be approved for surgery. Some patients thought the surgery would fix their health problems; others just wanted to look and feel better about themselves. As I gained more experience with these patients, I recognized the results were rarely what any patient truly wanted.

These are the three most common procedures: (1) the laparoscopic gastric banding (usually called the "lap band"), (2) the vertical sleeve gastrectomy (VSG), and (3) the Roux-en-Y gastric bypass (RYGB). Each has its own unique action on the body, but all three have some problems in common.

With the lap band procedure, a silicone ring is placed around the top portion of the stomach, known as the fundus. This creates a small pouch with an opening at the bottom for food and liquid to slowly leak into the rest of the stomach. The silicone ring has a

---

3   "Phentermine," *LiverTox*.
4   C. Seifarth, B. Scehler, and H. J. Schneider, "Effectiveness of Metformin on Weight Loss in Non-diabetic Individuals with Obesity," *Experimental and Clinical Endocrinology and Diabetes* 121, no. 1 (2012): 27–31, https://doi.org/10.1055/s-0032-1327734.

balloon that can be injected with saline from the outside of the body. When the balloon is inflated, the lap band causes the opening at the bottom of the pouch to be smaller. The person will consume less food and liquid and go longer between mealtimes because the lap band delays the emptying of food from the pouch into the remainder of the stomach.

Someone with a lap band is able to eat and drink only small amounts at a time, between ¼ and ¾ cup, depending on how much the balloon is inflated. When the lap band pouch is full, it produces pain, causing the person to stop eating. This occurs with a normal stomach as well; the fundus has nerve endings that signal pain when it is stretched, telling the brain the stomach is full and to stop eating or that food might come back up. The lap band creates a unique and unfortunate dilemma: the person continues to have all the normal hunger hormones secreted from the main portion of the stomach, but this person can eat only a small amount before the fullness pain returns. The individual is full and hungry at the same time, a confusing phenomenon for the body.

The vertical sleeve gastrectomy surgically alters the stomach. The surgeon removes most of the body of the stomach, leaving a small, banana-shaped stomach. Once again, this person can consume only a small amount of food or liquid at a time, around ½ cup after fully healed, leading to forced calorie reduction and therefore weight loss. By removing a significant portion of the stomach, a majority of the hormones responsible for signaling hunger are also removed.

The Roux-en-Y gastric bypass is more drastic than the VSG. Most of the stomach is cut away, leaving the person with a small pouch of stomach, referred to as the "remnant pouch." The remainder of the stomach is left inside the body along with the still-attached duodenum, the first third of the small intestine. The surgeon separates the duodenum from the jejunum, the second third of the small intestine, and attaches the jejunum to the remnant pouch. The end of the duodenum is then reattached to the jejunum but farther down. The result of the rearranged intestines is a Y formation. All this rearranging creates a digestive pathway that causes the small amount of food eaten to not be completely digested or absorbed by the body. A person who undergoes the RYGB experiences calorie restriction and also malabsorption of nutrients and calories, resulting in weight loss.

There are many downsides to each of these bariatric surgeries. The side effects common to all are nausea, vomiting, and dehydration. The VSG and RYGB also have the common side effect of dumping syndrome, a condition caused by consuming high-sugar or high-fat foods, which triggers blood sugar crashes and abdominal distress, typically leading to diarrhea, lightheadedness, nausea, vomiting, shakiness, sweating, flushing, or in more severe cases, loss of consciousness.

The more harmful side effect of these surgeries is malnutrition. I have seen many hospitalized patients who, earlier in life, had undergone bariatric surgery. These patients had obvious protein-calorie malnutrition as well as vitamin and mineral deficiencies. In fact, these deficiencies were likely the reason they were facing health problems.

One patient was a large woman in her mid-sixties who had undergone RYGB in her forties. She was admitted to the hospital for a broken hip. She told me she had a hard time eating enough at home. She admitted she never felt hungry and had to limit her food choices to prevent vomiting or diarrhea. She had talked to her doctor about these issues, but so far nothing had worked. She needed caregivers at home to help her shower and do her shopping and cooking because she always felt too weak. The day finally came when she got up to go to the bathroom and fell, breaking her hip. On my physical assessment, this woman had an obvious lack of muscle mass and strength, explaining her body weakness. She also reported not taking her vitamin D and calcium supplements for years, leading to deficiency and contributing to her weak bones.

Another case was a long-term care resident in the nursing home I worked at. She'd had a lap band for close to twenty years. A large, wheelchair-bound woman in her seventies, she had never been able to lose much weight with the lap band. What it did give her was gastrointestinal issues and a tolerance of only a limited selection of foods. She often was nauseous after eating and relied on antinausea meds to prevent vomiting. She couldn't eat meat or any raw fruits or vegetables because those foods felt "stuck" and usually made her throw up. She also had diabetes and avoided carbohydrates, thinking this would help her lose weight too. The telltale sign of her malnutrition came whenever she had wounds. Pressure sores (which are often caused by poor nutrition) on her backside took forever to heal. Her inadequate intake of calories, protein, vitamins, and minerals could be supplemented only so much. Whenever I recommended that she get the lap band removed, she declined. She still had hopes of one day using the forced restriction to help her lose weight, be mobile, and live on her own.

These bariatric surgeries too often put limitations on foods that can be consumed. I remember my patients especially missed traditional holiday foods, which were often high in fat or sugar. If they could eat them, it was just one small bite of everything before they were full. They were full physically but nowhere near satisfied. Sometimes patients would eat what or how much they wanted and just deal with the consequences. Other patients were not able to tolerate dairy after surgery, which previously had been a major source of calcium and protein in their diets.

As a dietitian working with bariatric surgery patients, I had to sign off that I felt the patient was nutritionally ready for surgery. Patients typically had four to six months of nutrition appointments with me, as required by their insurance company. I taught the Mediterranean diet, how to practice eating slowly and chew food well, how often to eat, which foods and beverages they would have to avoid, what foods cause dumping syndrome, how to drink liquids separate from eating food, how to incorporate exercise, which supplements they would require, and so on. I unfortunately saw many patients who really didn't want to change their behaviors and eating patterns. They believed they could implement change after surgery and be fine. There was pressure from the rest of the clinical team (and from the patient) for me to sign off on surgery even if I thought the patient was not ready. I often felt I was the only dietitian in the clinic who would put her foot down and require the patient to delay surgery until they could prove they were ready for the huge lifestyle change. It was a hard conversation to have with patients, and I often wondered if my patients lied to me, saying that they had changed their behaviors to get me to okay them for surgery.

Another problem I had with the program was the fact that they accepted adolescents. I occasionally had sixteen- or seventeen-year-old patients hoping to have bariatric surgery, which broke my heart. Their bodies were not done growing, and yet the surgeon, doctor, and parents thought it was okay to proceed with weight loss surgery. I worried about malnutrition and poor adherence to the lifelong changes that would be needed. Eventually, I was no longer assigned to these patients, as I strongly opposed them having the surgery.

Even adult patients struggled to continue following our nutrition advice after surgery. They would fall back into old habits, such as drinking soda. Or they would find foods they could get away with eating larger amounts of (such as soups or popcorn) so that they could keep eating when bored or for other emotional reasons. Sometimes patients would abuse alcohol when they couldn't tolerate the foods they once had been able to eat. I started to understand that surgery was not a guarantee for long-term weight loss. If their disordered eating had not been addressed before surgery, the same habits persisted, just changed to match their new circumstances. An altered stomach can eventually stretch out if the patient pushes the limit on how much they eat, and that patient can end up eating a normal amount of food again. Soon the weight they had lost would be regained. Some patients even had surgical revisions years after their original surgery.

The possibility of weight regain depends on the type of surgery the patient has had, but all have the potential for the patient to gain back the weight lost. In an article written for the *World Journal of Diabetes* in 2017, the authors state that patients with a lap band typically regain 35 percent to 40 percent of their lost weight. VSG patients have regained 5.7 percent of their lost weight at two years and as much as 75.6 percent of their lost weight at six years. Finally, for RYGB patients, 7 percent to 50 percent fail to maintain their weight loss.[5] A number of factors play into why weight regain occurs. As previously mentioned, the stomach may stretch out over time, allowing the person to eat more food. Or a person might not maintain a calorie deficit if they are consuming high-calorie foods or beverages, such as soda or alcohol. A theory gaining a lot of attention is that the depletion of lean body mass (muscle) that happens with all rapid weight loss causes the resting energy expenditure (REE, commonly referred to as a person's metabolism) to slow.[6] I will talk more about this concept in Chapter 3.

Patients were often disappointed that they did not lose as much weight as they had expected to. They wanted thin, perfect bodies. Most never got the perfect bodies they wanted, no matter how hard they tried. They never seemed to be satisfied with the amount of weight they lost. Once their weight plateaued, they panicked and asked for

---

5   Roberta Lupoli et al., "Bariatric Surgery and Long-Term Nutritional Issues," *World Journal of Diabetes* 8, no. 11 (2017): 464–74, doi:10.4239/wjd.v8.i11.464.
6   Charmaine S. Tam et al., "Energy Metabolic Adaptation and Cardiometabolic Improvements One Year After Gastric Bypass, Sleeve Gastrectomy, and Gastric Band," *The Journal of Clinical Endocrinology and Metabolism* 101, no. 1 (2016): 10, https://doi .org/10.1210/jc.2016-1814.

recommendations for how to lose more pounds. Many patients did not realize how much extra skin would be left after losing weight. Removing this loose skin is a whole other, expensive surgery that is not typically covered by insurance.

Luckily for me, as the program grew the two sides of the clinic split more definitively. This meant I did not have to see many patients pursuing surgery, as I was assigned to the medical weight loss program side. It was around this time that the clinic decided to start holding "lunch and learns" to expand our understanding of diets. We read books on mindful eating, functional nutrition, and elimination diets. Ironically enough, one of the books we read was *Intuitive Eating: A Revolutionary Program That Works*. In a better state of mind and with some experience under my belt, the IE research felt like a breath of fresh air. It was clear to me that dieting in the traditional sense of calorie deficit didn't work. No wonder so many of my patients struggled with losing weight and had a poor body image. But I didn't fully commit to the first principle of IE: reject the diet mentality. Part of me thought that intentional weight loss was still a possibility. I thought that if I could teach my patients to follow their hunger and fullness cues and fix their emotional eating, they could get to a "healthy weight," which in my mind meant a thinner body.

I started to change my tactics. Instead of giving my patients a calorie goal, I told them about intuitive eating (explained in detail in Chapter 4) and set-point weight theory (explained in Chapter 3). I told them to follow their body's hunger and fullness signals and they would eventually lose weight. But many of my patients were not invested in what I was telling them. They wanted calorie restriction because that had worked for them in the past. Many told me that their body was hungry all day. I explained that to fix their metabolism they needed to eat more, but that might cause initial weight gain. They didn't like to hear that, but I couldn't really blame them. They were coming to the clinic because they wanted to lose weight. Patients who did trust me enough to try IE sometimes ended up either staying the same weight or gaining weight, and they quickly gave up.

The next book our team read was *Health at Every Size*. Once again I was impressed by the anti-diet research, and by the time I finished the book, I realized I could no longer keep working at the clinic. I suddenly had an explanation for why my most challenging patients couldn't lose weight, and had labels for the negative self-talk that came from my patients: body image disorder, body dysmorphia, poor self-esteem, and poor self-image.

It depressed me to know that the reason most patients dieted was because they felt they needed to change how they looked to fit into Western society's idea of beautiful and healthy. I was burned out and ready to escape the world of weight loss.

As soon as the next job opportunity came along, I took it. My new job was at a skilled nursing facility, as far away from weight loss counseling as I could be—or so I thought. I should have realized that even outside a weight loss clinic, people would still be trying to lose weight, even people who had just been discharged from the hospital. Weight loss should have been the last thing on their minds. But when I introduced myself as the dietitian, patients of all sizes and weights typically either put up their guard because they thought I was going to tell them to lose weight or else peppered me with questions on how to lose weight.

Thankfully, my job rarely involved promoting weight loss. I was there to help these patients eat adequately and get stronger so they could go home. For patients who did want to talk about weight loss, I would answer their questions about which diets were really just fad diets and try to put them on the path of healthy eating. I wasn't an anti-diet dietitian yet. Although I loved the idea of HAES and IE, I hadn't quite accepted that a person shouldn't intentionally try to lose weight for health.

I did, however, see that weight stigma in health care was real. Doctors and nurse practitioners were the biggest culprits, although nurses and nursing assistants were quick to judge too. Assumptions were made about a patient's nutritional status based on their weight. Staff (without a nutrition degree, mind you) were having discussions with patients about their weight and how to eat healthier at home.

In one horrifyingly frustrating case, a patient weighed more than 300 pounds and was very sick. Only in her mid-thirties, this woman had destroyed her kidneys with drug use and was on hemodialysis treatment three or four times a week to stay alive. She also had large, nonhealing wounds on her abdomen. She was clearly depressed about her life. She was hardly eating and she slept a lot. Even at her size, she met the criteria for severe protein-calorie malnutrition. When I told this to the patient's nurse practitioner I was met with disagreement. The practitioner would not accept that the patient was malnourished and said, "She wouldn't be in this situation if she weren't so fat." Neither the practitioner nor the doctor would consider my argument to start tube feeding, a treatment that was highly indicated. Thankfully the dietitian at the dialysis center agreed that the patient was malnourished and provided her with additional intravenous nutrition during her dialysis treatments. In the end, it was not enough to keep her alive. She passed away in a few short weeks.

After leaving that job, I worked on call at a local hospital while starting up my private business. The weight bias there was even worse. The units I worked on were acute care and critical care. The biggest part of my job was to make recommendations to begin supplements, tube feeding, or intravenous nutrition for patients who were not eating enough (or at all). Many physicians would put off nutrition intervention with our larger patients, stating that they had adequate stores of nutrition, referring to their body fat.

In one instance, the patient was a large man in his forties placed in a medically induced coma and ventilated due to acute respiratory failure. The team was having difficulty weaning him from his coma due to continued agitation and combativeness. Treating ventilated patients can be tricky. Sometimes they wake up easily and other times it takes several days or longer. The standard practice is typically to start tube feeding or IV nutrition right away just in case it is the latter. But because of this patient's size, the doctors declined my recommendation to start tube feeding early. He went without a substantial amount of nutrition for four days. On the fifth day, I was allowed to start tube feeding through a tube that went from his mouth to his stomach. He was eventually weaned from the ventilator but continued to require tube feeding as he was not conscious enough to eat safely. The attending doctor agreed to have a feeding tube surgically placed into the patient's stomach, and we provided him nutrition this way for over a month. This therapy was lifesaving for this patient. Two months later he was able to be weaned from the tube feeding and discharged home eating a normal diet.

Maybe you are wondering, *Didn't he have enough stores to last a few days?* The answer is not straightforward. In times of severe, acute illness (think of a bad car crash or major surgery), the body is stressed. The metabolic rate rises as the body assesses its damage and starts the healing process. Without adequate calories or protein, the body turns to its own stores for fueling this process. The body will rapidly deplete the small amount of stored carbohydrates in the liver first. Then the body turns to fat and lean body mass (muscle) stores. The body is programmed to break down muscle more readily than fat for energy, although some fat is also converted to energy.[7]

So in the case of my patient, yes, he had some fat and muscle stores to live off of, but muscle should be preserved at all costs. We cannot simply tell the body to leave the muscle stores alone and pull only from fat stores for extra energy for healing. Research across the board shows that lower total lean body mass is the main factor in developing chronic disease; decreased strength, leading to disability and falls;[8] skin breakdown;[9] infection;[10] a prolonged recovery from illness; an increased length of hospital stay;[11] and so on. I've had to work hard to convince doctors and surgeons of this, sending them research articles and best practice recommendations. Still, many did not listen to reason or the research.

By this time, the fire in me was lit and raging. The mistreatment of people based solely on their size and not on their nutrition status (as determined by the experts) was maddening. I started to dig deeper into the research and pored over the teachings and work of my HAES colleagues. It was around this time that my brain finally was able to comprehend what diet culture was and what that meant. Diet culture was why my patients didn't get adequate treatment; why my hospitalized patients still wanted to lose weight (or, even worse, hoped they might lose weight because they were sick); why doctors recommended weight loss based on BMI; and why I had been so obsessed with having a flat tummy all those years. This realization was what inspired me to write this book. This is one way to tell the world that being a higher weight isn't a bad thing.

As my knowledge of Health at Every Size grew, the way I felt about my body started to change. I had gained weight after having my son and was aware that it was affecting me negatively. For a long time, I wore tummy control Spanx under my clothes to hide my stomach and back rolls. I begrudgingly gave away my old clothes, and the new ones I

---

7   Alfonso J. Cruz-Jentoft et al., "Sarcopenia: Revised European Consensus on Definition and Diagnosis," *Age and Ageing* 48, no. 1 (2019): 16–31, https://doi.org/10.1093/ageing/afy169.

8   Cruz-Jentoft et al., "Sarcopenia," 17, 23.

9   Jaul, E., J. Barron, J.P. Rosenzweig, and J. Menczel. "An Overview of Co-morbidities and the Development of Pressure Ulcers among Older Adults." *BMC Geriatrics* 18, no. 1 (2018). https://doi.org/10.1186/s12877-018-0997-7.

10   Nelke, C., R. Dziewas, J. Minnerup, S.G. Meuth, and T. Ruck. "Skeletal Muscle as Potential Central Link Between Sarcopenia and Immune Senescence." *EBioMedicine*, 49 (2019): 381–388. https://doi.org/10.1016/j.ebiom.2019.10.034.

11   Sousa, A., R. Guerra, I. Fonseca, I. et al. "Sarcopenia and Length of Hospital Stay." *European Journal Clinical Nutrition* 70, (2016): 595–601. https://doi.org/10.1038/ejcn.2015.207.

bought were oversized and hid my figure. I scolded myself for not being able to control my evening snacking.

Learning that weight was something I had little control over allowed me to finally let go of the suffocating reins. I stopped counting calories. I stopped fearing sugar. I stopped guilting myself for not exercising more. I began to embrace my curves and speak out against fatphobia. In practicing intuitive eating, I honored my hunger and fullness better; moved my body when it felt good to; and let go of the thoughts that certain foods were hurting me.

Little by little, food became pleasurable again. I allowed myself to explore my food preferences and rediscover what foods I liked. I went through the "honeymoon phase" of intuitive eating and allowed myself to eat all the foods that I had guilt-tripped myself about. Nowadays I sometimes have a hard time deciding what I want to eat because I have an abundance of the foods I like available.

Intuitive eating doesn't have a finish line. I've learned body acceptance and trust is about the journey. There are hills and valleys, easier days and harder days. I have to remind myself that my food choices or my body size are not the only things I want to spend my time thinking about. There is so much I want to accomplish and only one lifetime allotted. I hope by reading what I've learned, you can come to the same realization too.

Chapter 2

Health, BMI, and the Weight Loss Industry

Health is a subjective measure. Some think it is the absence of disease. Others say health is having a body that allows you to live the way you want to. Yet others say health means that you eat only nutritious foods and exercise daily. Most of Western society associates being thin with healthy, and therefore fat with unhealthy. The World Health Organization (WHO) defines health as "a state of complete physical, mental and social well-being and not merely the absence of disease or infirmity." So does body size have anything to do with health? Let's explore that question together in this chapter.

A brief history lesson: In 1998, the National Institutes of Health (NIH) held a conference to decide whether they should change the body mass index (BMI) standards to fall in line with the WHO's definitions. BMI is calculated using a person's weight and height. Research at the time indicated that a higher BMI was *not* correlated with a greater incidence of death.[12] In fact, the opposite was true. A higher BMI, up to around 32, was associated with living a longer life than a so-called normal BMI. Perhaps, the conversation went, the normal BMI range should be raised to reflect this.

---

12   Glenn A. Gaesser, "Thinness and Weight Loss: Beneficial or Detrimental to Longevity?" *Medicine and Science in Sports and Exercise* 31, no. 8 (1999): 1118–28, https://doi.org/10.1097/00005768-199908000-00007.

But instead of raising the BMI ranges to match the research, the NIH board lowered them to what we currently see today:

BMI

Underweight: <18.5

Normal weight: 18.5–24.99

Overweight: 25–29.99

Obese: 30+

Most members of the NIH board making this decision had personal reasons not to follow the research. These members had financial ties to the weight loss industry, specifically pharmaceutical companies selling weight loss drugs. The only NIH member on the advisory panel to vote against lowering the BMI standards was Judy Stern, an obesity researcher at the University of California at San Diego. She argued that the other board members were misquoting the research when they said the mortality rate increased at a BMI of 25.[13] By lowering the BMI normal ranges, the NIH effectively increased the number of individuals who "needed to lose weight" by about 29 million people. Profits for the weight loss industry skyrocketed. People spent money on diet drugs; weight loss programs, such as Jenny Craig; doctor visits; bariatric surgery; nutrition supplements; and so on. At the end of 2020, twenty-two years later, the US weight loss industry was estimated to be worth $71.1 billion.

BMI is a simplistic calculation, not a good indicator of someone's health. As already mentioned, BMI is a comparison of weight with height. BMI alone cannot tell you how much exercise a person does, what they eat, their stress level, how well they sleep, their gut health, or even how they look physically. BMI doesn't tell you about a person's body composition, waist circumference, or bone structure.

To give you an example of how variable BMI can look, think of a five foot, nine inch, 190-pound person. The BMI is calculated to be 28 and this person would be labeled "overweight." This person could look a number of different ways, depending on their gender and body composition. Actor Tom Hardy, who plays the villain Bane in *The Dark*

---

13   Sally Squires, "About Your BMI (Body Mass Index)," *Washington Post*, June 4, 1998.

Knight Rises, fits these measurements. Singer-songwriter Adele (before her dramatic weight loss) also fits this picture. Both would be considered unhealthy, and both would be advised to lose weight if health was based on only this simplistic number.

The index was created by the Belgian mathematician and scientist Lambert Adolphe Jacques Quetelet in the 1800s. He used BMI (called the Quetelet Index at the time) for population studies. Without calculators or computers in that time, Quetelet used this simple equation to measure the degree of obesity for his studies.[14] He never intended BMI to be used as a tool to assess an individual's health status because it does not take into account the other important factors already mentioned. This is why classifying obesity as a disease is bogus.

The so-called "obesity epidemic" is an example of blatant weight stigma that portrays being fat as a disease, and gives the illusion that weight is something that can and should be controlled by the individual. An obesity epidemic implies that people are gaining more and more weight exponentially over the years. But the fact is that people are heavier by only 6.6 to 11 pounds on average (3 to 5 kilograms) compared to people alive from 1960 to 1994.[15] This is hardly cause for alarm. People just on the edge of being "overweight" or "obese" are pushed barely over the line into these categories with their 6.6- to 11-pound weight gain, and the various health departments and organizations can thus claim that obesity rates have "doubled" or "tripled."

This "epidemic" doesn't hold much value unless there is a health danger tied to it, which is why the WHO claims that mortality rate increases with overweight or obese BMIs. Once again, these claims are overdramatized and poorly supported by research. Katherine Flegal is an epidemiologist, researcher, and consulting professor at Stanford University's Prevention Research Center. She is known for making a strong case in her research reviews that BMI is not associated with mortality.

Flegal uses a standard hazard ratio (HR) to predict all-cause mortality. A hazard ratio is a measure of the likelihood that someone will die at a given point as a result of being in

---

14   Keith Devlin, "Top 10 Reasons Why the BMI Is Bogus," *NPR*, July 4, 2009, https://www.npr.org/templates/story/story .php?storyId=106268439.

15   Lily O'Hara and Jane Taylor, "What's Wrong with the 'War on Obesity'? A Narrative Review of the Weight-Centered Health Paradigm and Development of the 3C Framework to Build Critical Competency for a Paradigm Shift," *SAGE Open* 8, no. 2 (2018), https://doi.org/10.1177/2158244018772888.

one group versus another. A baseline group has a hazard ratio of 1. If the comparison group has a hazard ratio greater than 1, group members are this much more likely to die because they are members of the group. The same goes for members of the comparison group if it has a hazard ratio of less than 1. Members are this much more likely *not* to die because they are members of the group. For example, if taking drug Y has a hazard ratio of 2 compared with the placebo group (HR = 1), you would be twice as likely to die from taking this drug. If the hazard ratio of drug Y is 0.5, you would be *half* as likely to die from taking this drug. This would be a good drug to take!

In Flegal's 2013 meta-analysis, she found that people with an "overweight" BMI had a hazard ratio of 0.94. This means people in this BMI category had a significantly lower risk of death overall compared with their normal BMI counterparts. People with a BMI of 30 to 34.9 (termed "class I obesity") had a hazard ratio of 0.95 compared with the normal BMI group. Once again, class I obesity had a lower risk of death than the normal BMI category.[16]

The last group, classes II and III obesity (BMI 35+) had a hazard ratio of 1.29 compared with the normal BMI group (that is, a 29 percent increase in the likelihood of death). Although this is significant, compare it with the hazard ratio of cigarette smoking (nondaily smokers HR 1.72, daily smokers HR 2.5, which is a 72 percent increase and a 250 percent increase in death risk, respectively).[17] Flegal's research supports many other studies and analyses, which come to similar conclusions.

Many studies that support a positive relationship between BMI and death do not account for significant confounding factors in their subjects, such as fitness level, diet quality, weight cycling, use of diet drugs, socioeconomic status, experienced weight stigma, or family history. Any of these factors mentioned could be possible reasons why a higher-weight individual has an increased risk of disease or death. Studies that do control for some of these factors often use self-reported data, jeopardizing the reliability and consequently the

16   Katherine M. Flegal et al., "Association of All-Cause Mortality with Overweight and Obesity Using Standard Body Mass Index Categories: A Systematic Review and Meta-analysis," *The Journal of the American Medical Association* 309, no. 1 (2013): 72–82, https://doi.org/10.1001/jama.2012.113905.
17   Maki Inoue-Choi et al., "Non-daily Cigarette Smokers: Mortality Risks in the United States," *American Journal of Preventive Medicine* 56, no. 1 (2019): 27–37, https://doi.org/10.1016/j.amepre.2018.06.025.

conclusions of these studies.[18] None of these studies can say with 100 percent certainty that a higher BMI or even a higher percentage of fat in body composition is the cause of death and disease, because *association* does not equal *causation*. It is also important to question whether these studies have been funded by or have a relationship with pharmaceutical or diet-selling companies. There have been multiple accounts of research conclusions being skewed in order to support the claim that being fat is unhealthy. The health care and weight management world does not like the research of Flegal and her colleagues because it threatens revenue.

Weight Stigma in Health Care

Weight stigma or bias comes in many forms, but in health care it can be quite serious. Doctors are often considered to be the biggest perpetrators of weight bias, but nurses, dietitians, therapists, social workers, nursing assistants, and other ancillary staff can stigmatize weight as well.[19] When weight bias is felt, stress and other negative emotions are created. At the weight loss clinic, there were many times when patients broke down crying after I asked my first question: "What brings you to the clinic?" Patients would tell me they were incredibly fearful of developing diabetes or dying young, which was what their doctors had told them could occur. Other patients were angry because they needed knee surgery but had to live with pain because the surgeon had told them they must lose weight first. All were frustrated. Rare was the patient who had not spent much of their lifetime trying to control their weight.

My point of view as a health care provider seeing weight stigma is also informed by my experience as a patient. In the recent past, I was on the receiving end of the "weight talk." I had made an appointment to be seen at a walk-in clinic for a urinary tract infection. I knew exactly what it was, and my attempts at home treatment had failed. It was time to get antibiotics. I did the normal song and dance with the medical assistant: I got weighed, she took my vitals, and then she asked about my reason for coming in. When the doctor arrived, he reviewed my symptoms and agreed I needed antibiotics. I thought I was good

18   Paul Campos et al., "The Epidemiology of Overweight and Obesity: Public Health Crisis or Moral Panic?" *International Journal of Epidemiology* 35, no. 1 (2006): 55–60, https://doi.org/10.1093/ije/dyi254.
19   Rebecca M. Puhl and Kelly D. Brownell, "Confronting and Coping with Weight Stigma: An Investigation of Overweight and Obese Adults," *Obesity* 14, no. 10 (2012): 1802–15, https://doi.org/10.1038/oby.2006.208.

to go—until he started talking to me about creating a healthy diet and exercise routine. He of course did not think to ask about my profession before launching into this talk. I wondered what exactly he was getting at, because I didn't think there was a diet or exercise that prevented UTIs. Finally, he let out the punch line: "Your BMI shows you are overweight, and you should think about trying to lose weight."

Flabbergasted is the only word to describe what I felt. My BMI was 25.1, barely inside the "overweight" classification. I'm also tall at five feet, ten inches, and my weight is pretty well distributed. My body had changed after having my son about a year prior, but I was by no means "unhealthy." The walk-in clinic doctor didn't think to ask me about my current diet and exercise habits, or medical history before launching into his speech. Because of my BMI, I got the "weight talk," which is dreaded by most people of size.

This weight lecture is based on the flawed research claims that a higher BMI causes worse health and a shorter life span. Doctors (and I would say most health care professionals) are educated all throughout their schooling on these claims. They are told it is their duty, according to their oath of "First do no harm," to talk to patients about their weight. But it is a dangerous speech in a number of ways.

First, it often makes the person feel ashamed and embarrassed about their size. The person may feel like a failure if they have tried to control their weight and were ultimately unsuccessful. Advising someone to lose weight adds another layer of stress, which we know is actually not good for health. Higher-weight individuals tend to experience chronic stress associated with weight bias, which is not limited to health care settings. People can experience weight bias from family or friends at home, work, school, or other social settings. The benefits of nutrition and exercise education may be negated when weight stigma is perceived, as this person will likely have irregular stress hormone regulation.[20] The body's inability to manage stress hormones effectively during an acutely stressful situation poses a risk to physical health. One way someone might cope with weight stigma is to just avoid places and situations where and when it can occur, including the doctor's office. They fear getting up on the too-small scale or needing the "special" larger blood pressure cuff. They worry that their medical concerns will not be fully heard or

---

20   Asia T. McCleary-Gaddy et al., "Weight Stigma and Hypothalamic–Pituitary–Adrenocortical Axis Reactivity in Individuals Who Are Overweight," *Annals of Behavioral Medicine* 53, no. 4 (2019): 392–98, https://doi.org/10.1093/abm/kay042.

addressed. So chronic health issues fester, and treatment of new issues are delayed or avoided altogether, as in the following example.

> Sarah had been diagnosed with type 2 diabetes a year prior. She had worked with a dietitian and an endocrinologist for about six months, and things were going well. She had lost some weight during those six months but had started to regain it. She was disappointed in herself and didn't want to face her medical team and tell them about the weight regain. She decided to wait until she lost the weight again before going back. Unfortunately, everything she tried eventually failed. She put off her appointments for more than a year because she knew (but also feared) what they would say. As a result, Sarah's blood sugars were even more out of control, and she fell further off her diabetes diet. By the time she finally went back to see the doctor, her blood sugar control was worse than when she had been diagnosed. Sarah was chastised by her doctor for not taking better care of her diabetes and controlling her weight. Sarah never went back to that doctor again.

Often medical providers do not listen to or treat health issues the same across weight classes. Larger people are often told their health issues are weight related, and weight loss is prescribed as the first line of treatment. Research shows that physicians choose to spend less time with higher weight individuals (likely due to stereotyping fat people as weak-willed or lazy), and often standard tests are not run, which leads to a delay in disease diagnosis and treatment.[21, 22] A larger person has a greater propensity for advanced disease states and worse health outcomes due to stigma-related misdiagnosis and a lack of effective treatment.[23]

Following is James's story—one example, out of who knows how many—that shows how deadly weight stigma in health care can be.

---

21 Gary D. Foster et al., "Primary Care Physicians' Attitudes About Obesity and Its Treatment." *Obesity Research* 11, no. 10 (2012): 1168–77, https://doi.org/10.1038/oby.2003.161.

22 Jennifer A. Lee and Cat J. Pause, "Stigma in Practice: Barriers to Health for Fat Women," *Frontiers in Psychology* 7 (2016): 2063, https://doi.org/10.3389/fpsyg.2016.02063.

23 S. M. Phelan et al., "Impact of Weight Bias and Stigma on Quality of Care and Outcomes for Patients with Obesity," *Obesity Reviews* 16, no. 4 (2015): 319–26, https://doi.org/10.1111/obr.12266.

James complained of chronic, debilitating bone pain. Think of growing pains when you were a kid, but at least ten times worse and nonstop. James voiced this to his doctor at every appointment. And every time he was told that he just needed to lose weight.

James was a large man, around six foot, four inches and very heavyset. He had dieted for most of his adult life, but every attempt to diet now in his late fifties was futile. He had no desire to move due to his pain, but he did his best to eat "healthy" and go for short walks. His weight never budged. He tried other methods to relieve the pain, such as massage and acupuncture, but had no luck. Finally, James decided to get a second and even a third opinion. His newest doctor talked with him about his health history, and when she discovered that James had a history of cancer, she immediately ordered blood tests and scans. Sure enough, James had been walking around with stage III bone cancer for nearly two years.

Weight stigma also has an impact on mental health. It is estimated that 40 percent of higher weight people have internalized weight bias, meaning they are aware of the negative stereotype associated with their identity, they agree with the stereotype and apply it to themselves, and as a result, experience self-devaluation. Internalized weight bias has been associated with depression, anxiety, emotional distress, poor self-esteem, body dissatisfaction and body image concerns, disordered eating and eating disorder pathology (such as binge eating disorder and bulimic symptoms), and psychological distress.[24, 25] Research also indicates that people who perceive discrimination in the form of weight stigma are 2.5 times as likely to develop mood or anxiety disorders and have a higher risk of developing depression.[26]

Weight stigma is demoralizing. It demotivates someone to develop healthy eating habits or exercise for their health. When a person experiences weight stigma, they are saddled with stress, putting them at greater risk for physical or mental illness. We must stop

---

24   R. L. Pearl and R. M. Puhl, "Weight Bias Internalization and Health: A Systematic Review," *Obesity Reviews* 19, no. 8 (2018): 1141–63, https://doi.org/10.1111/obr.12701.

25   Phelan et al., "Impact of Weight Bias."

26   Janet A. Tomiyama et al., "How and Why Weight Stigma Drives the Obesity 'Epidemic' and Harms Health," *BMC Medicine* 16, no. 123 (2018), https://doi.org/10.1186/s12916-018-1116-5.

treating "obesity" as a disease and work on accepting that bodies are meant to be diverse in size and to change as we age and experience life. Weight change should be considered a symptom of or response to what is going on in the body. Weight gain is associated with the diseases of hypothyroidism and polycystic ovary syndrome, but weight gain doesn't always indicate something is wrong. For example, many researchers would like to know why young women in their twenties and early thirties tend to gain weight. They fear that if these women don't prevent weight gain, horrible ailments and chronic disease will befall them. Some hypothesize the weight gain is due to a lack of knowledge about nutrition, eating too much or not eating the "right" foods (for example, "giving in to" premenstrual cravings), or not exercising enough. But isn't it logical to hypothesize that the female body is naturally trying to situate itself for optimal health during its childbearing years? Is it so far-fetched to think that this natural, amazing thing our bodies can do is actually a good thing? Is it incomprehensible that we are not supposed to remain in our adolescent-size bodies our whole lives? Weight isn't something that can easily be controlled, a thought that is inconsistent with what our society wants us to believe. In Chapter 3, you'll discover why intentional weight loss is so often impossible and how it can actually be worse for your health.

Chapter 3

How the Body Responds to Intentional Weight Loss

Dieting and weight loss are common recommendations in health care, but are never discussed in the way that other treatment options or procedures are. When a doctor discusses starting a new medication, the benefits are explained as well as the potential side effects and risks. If a doctor were to discuss the risks and benefits of starting a diet, I doubt anyone would agree to it. To begin, multiple studies indicate that fewer than 5 percent of dieters are able to lose even 5 percent of their weight and keep it off for two years.[27] Roughly 80 percent of people who intentionally achieve a weight loss of 10 percent or more will regain that weight within a year.[28] A treatment option with a failure rate of 95 percent or more isn't an effective treatment.

---

27   D. Crawford, R. W. Jeffery, and S. A. French, "Can Anyone Successfully Control Their Weight? Findings of a Three Year Community-Based Study of Men and Women," *International Journal of Obesity* 24 (2000): 1107–10, https://doi.org/10.1038/sj.ijo.0801374.

28   Alison Feldes et al., "Probability of an Obese Person Attaining Normal Body Weight: Cohort Study Using Electronic Health Records," *American Journal of Public Health* 105, no. 9 (2015): e54–59, https://doi.org/10.2105/AJPH.2015.302773.

Although doctors are perceived as the highest authority in health care, they typically have little education when it comes to nutrition. Whom would you prefer advising you about nutrition: a doctor, who has spent on average 19.6 hours studying nutrition,[29] or a registered dietitian, who has spent a minimum of three years studying nutrition? Doctors are the most weight-stigmatizing practitioners and yet are the least educated in how food and exercise play into weight control and metabolism.

This dangerous combination didn't play out well for one patient of mine: a man in his mid-forties, who ended up in the hospital because of the diet his doctor had prescribed for him, the well-known ketogenic (keto) diet. This higher-weight patient had been following the keto diet for about three months before extreme abdominal pain set in. At the hospital, he was found to be in liver failure and underwent an emergent exploratory laparotomy. He spent the next four weeks recovering from his major surgery and liver failure at the skilled nursing facility, trying to work from a laptop in his hospital bed.

Diet prescription is a complicated treatment option and should not be attempted by just anyone, including doctors, self-proclaimed nutritionists, and personal trainers. There is no one-size-fits-all eating plan that will make everyone healthy or conform to one body size. Humans are diverse in size and shape, just like we are diverse in eye color and height. Your body is so amazing and smart that it will do exactly what is right to protect you and keep you thriving.

To help you understand why intentional weight loss is harmful, let's talk through how the human body and brain react in response to dieting. Think of this as the full disclosure of the "risk" side of the weight loss risk–benefit analysis. Here is a true account, so common it might as well be in a textbook, to help you better understand these risks:

> Beth had watched her mom diet for as long as she could remember. When she was eleven, Beth was put on her first diet. Puberty had been changing her body: her breasts were growing larger, her hips were widening, and she was a little thicker around her middle. Beth wasn't great about following her diet. Her mom

---

29   David J. Frantz et al., "Current Perception of Nutrition Education in U.S. Medical Schools," *Current Gastroenterology Reports* 13 (2011): 376–79, https://doi.org/10.1007/s11894-011-0202-z.

prepared and portioned out all her food at home, but at school Beth used her own money to buy pizza and other snacks from the cafeteria.

Her body continued to fill out in her preteen years, and as a freshman in high school, Beth started getting comments on her body from her peers. She was called "fat" or "pig" during lunch hour at school. It didn't help that her mom reflected those comments at home and continued to push low-calorie food. Beth decided it was time to take weight loss more seriously. She exercised in the school gym during her lunch instead of eating, and she started following her mom's dieting advice. They even bonded over their dieting experience.

Beth started to lose weight and was highly praised by her mother and friends. When summer came the school gym was closed, and Beth's exercise routine abruptly ended. With no structured exercise routine and some eating out of boredom, Beth ended up regaining all the weight—and 5 pounds more. Feeling defeated, she tried again to lose weight.

We will continue Beth's story as we go through the body's response to dieting and intentional weight loss. We first must talk about the concept of a calorie deficit. Although cleverly disguised in phrases such as "portion control" or "eat less, move more," a calorie deficit is the basis for almost every diet plan, including Beth's diets. A calorie is a measurement of energy, so we could also call a calorie deficit an "energy deficit."

To achieve a calorie deficit, one must create an energy imbalance in the body. The resting metabolic rate (RMR), which is sometimes called the basal metabolic rate (BMR), is the energy the body uses *at rest*; it is the energy needed to keep the heart pumping, the lungs inflating, and so on. On average, the RMR accounts for 60 percent of the body's daily energy expenditure.[30] To simplify this concept, think of the RMR as the body's metabolism. To create an energy deficit, a person can (1) eat fewer calories or (2) exercise in order to burn internal calories, or internal energy stores, for energy. Usually a person trying to lose weight does some combination of both.

---

30   John W. Pelley, "Nutrition," chapter 19, in *Elsevier's Integrated Review Biochemistry*, 2nd ed. (2012): 171–79, https://doi .org/10.1016/B978-0-323-07446-9.00019-2.

Left to its own devices, the body has a certain weight it likes to hover around, based on its individual metabolism. In the health world, this is called the *set-point weight theory*.[31] Calorie deficit diets are a way to intentionally lower body weight. When the body doesn't get enough calories through food, or must use extra calories for exercise, it will start using its internal energy stores (what most people assume are going to be their fat stores) to make up the extra calories needed to support the set-point weight. Eventually, as the body uses up its own energy stores and they are not replaced with enough external calorie intake (food), weight loss is induced.

Although that might seem fine and dandy, the body systems are processing this negative energy imbalance in a much different way. Our bodies are designed for self-preservation in all circumstances. If they weren't, humans as a species would have died out a long time ago. In the setting of inadequate food (calorie) intake, the body shifts into protection mode (some refer to this as starvation mode). Even though the eyes can see that there is plenty of food in the refrigerator or cupboards, the brain and body process the decreased calorie intake to mean, *There must not be enough food around. We will starve!*

The brain starts to make food a top priority. Thoughts about food are more frequent than they were before. Hunger pangs are stronger as the body tries to signal it is missing those calories normally eaten. A person might feel faint, nauseous, or lethargic when restricting calorie intake. Although fat may be the most abundantly stored energy source for some bodies, metabolically, it is the hardest for the body to convert to energy. This means the body will exhaust other available sources of fuel before turning to the fat stores.

The body will first use up any carbohydrate stores. The body relies on daily carbohydrate consumption, which it breaks down to glucose via digestion. Glucose is used by all body cells for energy. The brain and a few other body tissues use glucose exclusively for energy and will not accept other sources. Even though carbs are necessary for our existence, little glucose is stored in the body. When the body is unable to obtain glucose from the food you eat, the body will make glucose out of the body's store of amino acids. When

31 Richard E. Keesey and Matt D. Hirvonen, "Body Weight Set-Points: Determination and Adjustment," *Journal of Nutrition* 127, no. 9 (1997): 1875S–83S, https://doi.org/10.1093/jn/127.9.1875S.

you eat protein foods, the body digests them down to amino acids. The body typically uses amino acids to build muscle but can also use them to make glucose. The body is not above reaping amino acids from your own muscles to make glucose when an inadequate amount of carbohydrates or protein are eaten. This is a detrimental consequence of losing weight. Muscle mass plays a big part in metabolism. A greater muscle mass is associated with a higher metabolism (which explains why men are generally able to lose weight easier than can women, who typically have a greater fat mass compared with muscle mass). Of course, a greater muscle mass means greater strength, endurance, and balance, all of which are needed to do the activities of daily living, such as climbing stairs or mowing the lawn. People with a lower percentage of body muscle mass are at increased risk of falls or disability, a reduced quality of life, and an increased chance of disease or death.[32]

In the starvation response, the body must still preserve essential muscles, such as heart muscle. At a certain point, the body will turn to the last available energy source, the fat stores, also called lipids. After about three days of inadequate carbohydrate intake, the body starts to make ketone bodies from stored lipids.[33] I bet you're thinking, *Where have I heard that word* ketone *before?* A ketone is what is produced in the process of ketogenesis. The popular diet known as the ketogenic diet, or keto diet, takes advantage of this process. Ketones are a last-resort, alternative energy source the body can make when inadequate glucose is available. A body in a calorie deficit will use a combination of glucose (when it's available or from muscle stores) and ketones produced to meet its energy needs.

The keto diet is my least favorite fad diet as it makes carbohydrates, which are needed by *every* body, out to be poisonous. There is not much known about the long-term effects of being in ketosis. We do know that the liver works hard to produce the amount of ketones needed to keep a person alive while the body is in ketosis. There is research showing that the keto diet can lead to fatty liver, kidney stones, ketoacidosis, and potentially death.[34]

---

32 Josep M. Argilés et al., "Skeletal Muscle Regulates Metabolism via Interorgan Crosstalk: Roles in Health and Disease," *Journal of Post-acute and Long-Term Care Medicine* 17, no. 9 (2016): 789–96, https://doi.org/10.1016/j.jamda.2016.04.019.

33 Jeremey M. Berg, John L. Tymoczko, and Lubert Stryer, "Food Intake and Starvation Induce Metabolic Changes," in *Biochemistry*, 5th ed. (New York: W. H. Freeman and Company, 2002).

34 James McIntosh, "What to Know About Ketosis," *Medical News Today*, 2020, https://www.medicalnewstoday.com/articles/180858.

As the days and weeks of the calorie deficit go on, the body's metabolism slows in an effort to preserve energy and body weight.[35] This can worsen the dieter's tiredness, grumpiness, weakness, and lack of concentration. Although a few pounds have been lost, the body is far from feeling healthy. Eventually, the metabolism slows to a point where a calorie deficit is no longer achievable. Let's continue Beth's story:

> At twenty-five, Beth was frustrated with her weight. She had tried many diets over the past fourteen years and had finally decided to get professional help. Her primary doctor referred her to a dietitian, who calculated her RMR with a predictive equation known as the Harris-Benedict equation. The dietitian gave Beth a calorie goal of 1,650 calories per day and told her to track her food and exercise in a fitness app. She also gave her lists of foods she should and shouldn't eat.
>
> Finally, the scale started to show weight loss again. Beth steadily lost 2 to 5 pounds a week for two months. Then the weight loss slowed; she was losing only 1 pound a week. Then 1 pound every two weeks. She tried bumping up her exercise and cutting her calories more, but lost only 2 pounds that month. And then, without Beth changing her routine at all, the weight loss stopped.
>
> The dietitian tried to encourage her, saying that the plateau wouldn't last. Beth just had to keep it up, and eventually the numbers on the scale would start moving down again. But instead the opposite happened. After being at the plateau for two weeks, the scale showed Beth was gaining weight.

At this point, Beth's metabolism had slowed in an effort to protect her. The body wants to stay at its set-point weight, the weight at which the body is happy, and will drop the metabolic rate lower to prevent further weight loss. Beth's weight plateau means her RMR had slowed enough to match her calorie intake. She was unable to burn enough calories through exercise or eat so few calories that she could get back into an energy deficit. When she started to gain weight, her metabolism had slowed enough to put her

---

35 A. G. Dulloo, J. Jacquet, and J-P Montani, "Pathways from Weight Fluctuations to Metabolic Diseases: Focus on Maladaptive Thermogenesis During Catch-Up Fat," *International Journal of Obesity*, no. 26 (2002): S46–57, https://doi.org/10.1038/sj.ijo.0802127.

into calorie excess (even though she was eating only 1,300 to 1,500 calories a day at that point).

Disappointed that she had failed at weight loss again, Beth quit going to the dietitian. She was tired of feeling hungry and mentally exhausted. What was the point of continuing the diet when she was gaining weight anyway? That week Beth ate everything she had been craving for the past few months. She ate every meal until she felt stuffed. She felt out of control with her eating. She avoided the scale, not wanting to face the numbers, which she knew were climbing.

Fast-forward ten years. Beth was now thirty-five and the heaviest she had ever been. She had continued to ride the roller coaster of weight loss–weight gain for the past ten years and had tried every diet known to man. The dieting attempts didn't last nearly as long as they once had. Binge eating broke her diet every time. And started it actually; when she was about to begin a new diet, she ate all the "bad" foods she wanted until the new diet commenced.

She decided enough was enough: it was time to get the weight off for good. She made an appointment with a weight loss doctor. The clinic performed a test called indirect calorimetry, a way of measuring the resting metabolic rate with good accuracy compared with the predictive equations typically used. The numbers were disappointing. Beth's RMR was about 400 calories per day lower than the average for a woman of her age.

The doctor prescribed the following plan: eat 1,000 calories daily and burn 500 calories daily in exercise to get to the calorie deficit needed to induce weight loss. He also advised her to consider bariatric surgery, as it would be difficult for her to maintain this strict diet for the long term. Beth left the clinic feeling hopeless and unsure of what to do next.

Beth's metabolism was slow due to her many attempts at weight loss. The process of weight cycling (the weight gain–weight loss roller coaster) changes the body composition toward more fat[36] and less lean body mass (muscle).[37] Every time Beth quit her diet and ate what she wanted again, her body used many of those new calories to replace her fat stores, and it added additional pounds of fat to protect her, ensuring she had enough energy stores for the next time she was starving, that is, dieting. This is the biggest reason dieters gain more pounds than they lose. Even more troubling is the fact that Beth's lean body mass never had a chance to recover. Building muscle is a slow process and takes a lot of nourishment. Beth's metabolism will remain low unless she stops dieting for good.

Weight cycling has dangerous implications. Research shows that people who yo-yo diet and weight cycle increase their risk of eating disorders; psychological disorders, such as anxiety or depression; type 2 diabetes and insulin resistance; dyslipidemia; high blood pressure; cardiovascular disease; cancer; bone fractures; and death.[38, 39, 40] More likely than not, Beth is malnourished. Eating so few calories over the years, she has been unable to consume adequate vitamins and minerals. She also likely has sarcopenic obesity, a disease characterized by high fat mass and low muscle mass, which puts a person at risk for disease, disability, falls, hospitalization, and death.[41]

Are you starting to rethink your desire to lose weight yet? Do you need more evidence that calorie deficit diets are dangerous? The Minnesota Starvation Experiment is a famous study conducted from 1944–1945. The deprivation experienced by many during World War II raised questions about how to renourish a person who has experienced extreme starvation. The primary researcher, Ancel Keys, recruited young, healthy male volunteers to endure semistarvation (calorie deficit) for six months, and then he studied the best ways of refeeding them.

At the start of the semistarvation period, the men were instructed to lose 2.5 pounds per week, with the goal of losing 25 percent of their total body weight by the end of

36 Philippe Jacquet et al., "How Dieting Might Make Some Fatter: Modeling Weight Cycling Toward Obesity from a Perspective of Body Composition Autoregulation," *International Journal of Obesity*, no. 44 (2020): 1243–53, https://doi.org/10.1038/s41366-020-0547-1.

37 Dulloo, "Pathways from Weight Fluctuations."

38 Dulloo, "Pathways from Weight Fluctuations."

39 J-P Montani, Y. Schutz, and A. G. Dulloo, "Dieting and Weight Cycling as Risk Factors for Cardiometabolic Diseases: Who Is Really at Risk?" *Obesity Reviews* 16, no. 1 (2015): 7–18, https://doi.org/10.1111/obr.12251.

40 Gaesser, "Thinness and Weight Loss."

41 Kyung Mook Choi, "Sarcopenia and Sarcopenic Obesity," *The Korean Journal of Internal Medicine* 31, no. 6 (2016): 1054–60, https://doi.org/10.3904/kjim.2016.193.

the starvation period. They were allotted 1,800 calories per day and required to walk 22 miles per week. From week to week the food portions changed for each participant, depending on whether the participant was meeting the goal weight loss rate. Ultimately, thirty-two volunteers completed the groundbreaking study. Here are some highlights from the article "They Starved So That Others Be Better Fed: Remembering Ancel Keys and the Minnesota Experiment" by Leah M. Kalm and Richard D. Semba.[42]

- The men had low energy and were weak. One man recalled having to wait outside a library until someone else opened the big door because he lacked the strength to open it. Another recalled that he had memorized where all the elevators were in buildings he frequented.

- Minute things annoyed the men; they became easily irritated at one another, especially about eating habits.

- The men experienced physical symptoms: dizziness, muscle soreness, hair loss, intolerance of the cold (even in summer months), reduced coordination, and ringing in the ears. Of course their appearance changed as well. They had sunken faces, protruding bones, and swollen legs, ankles, and faces.

- All the men had an obsession with food. Some would hold their food in their mouths for a long time to savor it and make the meal last longer. Others would dilute their food with water to make it look like a bigger meal. Food was constantly on their minds. One participant reported going to the movies and was more interested in what the actors were eating than the film itself.

- They were apathetic and lethargic, with no interest in dating or sex.

- The men referred to their diet as a religion of sorts, and felt that keeping on the diet was a dedication to their faith.

- When rehabilitation started, many men said they felt no relief. Even those eating 4,000 calories a day still experienced hunger.

---

42   Leah M. Kalm and Richard D. Semba, "They Starved So That Others Be Better Fed: Remembering Ancel Keys and the Minnesota Experiment," *The Journal of Nutrition* 135, no. 6 (2005): 1347–52, https://doi.org/10.1093/jn/135.6.1347.

- After completing the three-month rehabilitation, the men did not feel back to normal. Some men were physically ill (and one was hospitalized) from eating so much. They could not satisfy their cravings for food just by filling their stomachs.

I encourage you to read this fascinating research. Although the study was conducted more than seventy-five years ago, it is still relevant because human biology and physiology have not changed. Many of the issues summarized in the preceding list happen to people with disordered eating behaviors. Chronic dieters are known for being grumpy or irritable when restricting calories or certain foods. Losing hair, feeling cold all the time, and having little energy are also dieting hallmarks. Even though this study was about an extreme diet, people follow very low calorie diets every day (and some with even more restrictions). Think of Beth's last diet prescription: eat 1,000 calories per day and burn 500 calories in exercise daily. Although this calorie deficit most likely does not cause Beth to look like the emaciated men in the starvation study, she is malnourished.

Many people who intentionally lose weight meet the criteria for malnutrition as proposed by the American Society for Parenteral and Enteral Nutrition (ASPEN) and the Academy of Nutrition and Dietetics.[43] A few of the main components of malnutrition that are commonly seen in dieters are inadequate energy intake (as determined by a medical professional, typically a dietitian), significant weight loss within a defined time frame, depletion of lean body mass or fat mass, and loss of functional strength.

During her medically prescribed diet at age twenty-five, Beth could be classified as acutely malnourished because she (1) lost more than 5 percent of her body weight in one month, (2) consumed less than 75 percent of her estimated energy needs, and (3) had a moderate loss of lean body mass and fat mass. But instead of being cautioned that she was losing weight too quickly, she was praised for her weight loss efforts.

Few health care providers are trained to recognize the signs and symptoms of disordered eating or an eating disorder. An even smaller number of these providers recognize when an eating disorder is present in a larger person. All too often, extreme weight

---

43 "Table: Academy of Nutrition and Dietetics (Academy)/American Society for Parenteral and Enteral Nutrition (ASPEN) Clinical Characteristics That the Clinician Can Obtain and Document to Support a Diagnosis of Malnutrition," *Journal of the Academy of Nutrition and Dietetics* 112, no. 5 (2012): 734–35, https://www.andeal.org/vault/2440/web/files/ONC/Table_Clinical%20 Characteristics%20to%20Document%20Malnutrition-White%20JV%20et%20al%202012.pdf.

loss measures are supported and encouraged by everyone in the dieter's life: medical professionals, family, friends, coworkers, peers, and so on. The importance is placed on being a "normal" weight, no matter what it takes.

This is the main reason why eating disorders and disordered eating behaviors all too often go unrecognized, undiagnosed, and untreated. Many of the chronic dieters I know do not even realize that their behaviors are causing them harm. For instance, Maxine was experimenting with intermittent fasting for weight loss, which had been recommended by her doctor. She ate only one or two meals per day and couldn't tell she was hungry unless she was ravenous. She was never told that she was eating too little to support good nutrition. Other dieters are very aware that their eating habits are a problem but don't know how to stop the repeating cycles. Take me, for instance. Earlier in life, I was trying to "be good" and eat healthy, thinking I would lose weight. In front of others I could control myself, but every evening at home, without fail, the cravings returned. I would eat "bad" snacks until bedtime. I hated that I did that and always vowed to do better the next day.

Eating behaviors like mine are often a secret. It is embarrassing to not be "in control" or to "lack willpower." The problem stems from the restriction. *The more that food is restricted, the more that you crave it.* When something is off-limits, that alone can make us want it all the more. It never crossed my mind to reach out for help with my binges. I didn't want anyone to know I felt out of control with food. Plus, I was supposed to be a nutrition expert. I remember telling patients who had the same excessive snacking dilemma to chew gum or keep their hands busy by coloring or knitting. My own advice didn't work for me. In reality, I was making our disordered eating worse by imposing restrictions on when and what we could eat.

Disordered eating and eating disorders are on the rise due to diet culture. Starting at a young age, we learn that thinness equals beauty and health. The media help to portray this. Advertisers use thin models. The main character of a movie is most likely thin, and a fat actor (if there is one) is portrayed as lazy, out of shape, unhygienic, uncoordinated, unhealthy, and ugly. He or she is often the butt of jokes (think of Kevin from *The Office* or Amy in *Pitch Perfect*). This is diet culture. We accept this stereotyping and as a result, create unattainable beauty standards, develop unnatural eating habits, and disconnect from our bodies.

Disordered eating or a disordered eating mindset is the gateway to a true eating disorder. Symptoms of an eating disorder are starting to show up in children at a much younger age.[44] What may start out as an innocent attempt to eat healthier or lose a few pounds can quickly turn into an unhealthy obsession with looks and health. In no way has an individual done something wrong because he or she does not have a perfect body. There is no way for a body to be wrong! There is, however, a problem with our culture.

Weight stigma also exists in the eating disorder treatment world. Although an eating disorder is recognized as a serious mental illness, medical professionals may use a person's BMI as the deciding factor in an eating disorder diagnosis: if the person has a "normal" BMI or greater, a diagnosis could be denied.[45] Insurance companies can deny coverage for eating disorder treatment, even with a diagnosis, if a person's BMI is not considered "underweight."[46] These factors play a huge role in whether someone struggling with an eating disorder can obtain and afford treatment, with higher-weight people less likely to get help.

Amanda Kieser struggles with this as a licensed mental health counselor associate (LMHCA) who works as a therapist at an inpatient eating disorder treatment center. She believes that using weight or BMI is an outdated method to determine someone's health. Kieser works with people of all shapes and sizes who want to improve their relationship with food and body. Like many Health at Every Size practitioners, she believes that diet culture has influenced everyone—and we must unlearn its harmful lessons.

In this chapter, we've discussed the biggest risks associated with intentional weight loss. Let's recap: dieting has a 95 percent or greater failure rate with a high likelihood of weight regain; can cause your body to go into starvation mode, which leads to body composition change towards greater fat mass and less muscle mass; can cause your metabolism to slow over time, resulting in weight cycling; can cause malnutrition; and

---

44   "Eating Disorder Statistics," *National Eating Disorders Association,* accessed July 6, 2021, https://www.nationaleatingdisorders .org/toolkit/parent-toolkit/statistics.
45   Lee and Pause, "Stigma in Practice."
46   "Getting Insurance Approval: Arguments to Support Your Claim," *National Eating Disorders Association,* accessed July 6, 2021, https://www.nationaleatingdisorders.org/getting-insurance-approval-arguments-support-your-claim.

can lead to disordered eating and poor mental health, which can ultimately turn into an eating disorder. Are the benefits of being thin really more significant than the risk of poor mental and physical health? Research shows that being a higher weight does not automatically mean a shorter life *and* that weight is something we have little control over. Let's move on to learning body acceptance, how to trust yourself around food, and what you can control when it comes to your health.

***

There is much more involved in the body's mental, hormonal, and metabolic processes when it experiences a calorie deficit than I can address in this book. If you'd like to know more, check out Appendix A on page 121 for books that go into depth on this process. You can also read my interview with Amanda Kieser in Appendix B to learn more about her role in treating eating disorders.

Chapter 4

No More Diets! So How Do I Eat Now?

By now you might have decided that purposeful weight loss isn't worth the effort. Diet culture plants the idea that a bigger body is a problem that needs to be fixed. Attempting to shrink the body, causes more harm than good. Thankfully there is another way for you to coexist with food. I want to acknowledge that it can be frightening to give up on weight loss. For your first journal entry, I want you to create space for your feelings about this. It's time to show yourself that dieting has not helped you in the least.

Describe your personal history with dieting. List all dieting attempts and how your weight changed with each. How has dieting affected your emotional/mental health, your relationships, your confidence, your financial health, and your physical health?

HOW I RELATE TO FOOD AND BODY QUIZ

It is always important to know where you stand in your journey to food freedom. This quiz can help you see where you are currently in your relationship with food and body. Indicate how often you do the following (daily, weekly, monthly, yearly, once in a lifetime, never):

Behavior/Feeling	Frequency
I avoid certain foods because they are too high in calories, fat, carbs, salt, sugar, and so on.	
I worry about how many calories are in the food I eat.	
I track my calories, macronutrients, or food intake down to the smallest bite.	
I tell myself I can't have certain foods because they are not good for me.	
I feel guilty after eating an "unhealthy" food.	
I choose not to go to social events because I feel out of control around all the food.	
I attempt to strictly follow a diet plan for what or when I am allowed to eat.	
I try to control my weight through food or exercise.	
I eat because I am stressed, angry, sad, or lonely.	
I eat because I am bored.	
I eat the entire thing without meaning to.	
I eat past comfortable fullness; I feel sick after I'm done eating.	
I feel guilty for eating a lot of food in one sitting.	
I eat too much and force myself to "make up" the calories through exercise.	
I eat too much and self-induce vomiting or take laxatives.	
I go too long without eating and then eat everything in sight.	

Behavior/Feeling	Frequency
I skip meals or go to bed hungry in hopes of losing weight.	
I have low self-esteem and confidence because of my body.	
I plan my future around when I lose weight.	
My thoughts about food and my body make me anxious or depressed.	

All these statements reflect disordered eating behaviors or a disordered eating mindset. For the statements that happen frequently, such as daily or weekly, spend a bit more time on the prompts or activities that help you restore balance to these areas. As you go through the workbook, remember to let your self-compassion voice reign in your thoughts. There is no shame in where you are starting this journey to healing and health. Diet culture is the cause of your learned food and body issues, *not* you!

In this chapter I share with you my passion for intuitive eating. I believe that intuitive eating is the best way to heal from diet culture. I summarize the ten principles of IE and then present the research supporting this non-diet approach. It is important that you find *your* way of nourishing and respecting your body. There is no way to do it wrong. And there is no need to compare yourself with someone else. It is your relationship with your own body that is in need of repair, and no one knows your body except you. So with that mindset, read on.

Unfortunately, the terms *mindful eating* and *intuitive eating* have been incorporated into diet culture. Although these terms are not interchangeable, to become an intuitive eater, you need mindfulness. As more people latch onto the anti-diet approach, diet culture scrambles to find ways to stay relevant to us. For example, there is the "hunger-fullness" diet, which claims to be IE but says that a person will lose weight if they eat just when they are hungry, and stop when they are full. Even the Noom app claims to incorporate IE, but still has you track food and calories and promotes itself as a weight loss app. Do not be fooled: a diet is a diet.

Intuitive eating is very much *not* a diet. Evelyn Tribole and Elyse Resch, authors of the book *Intuitive Eating: A Revolutionary Anti-Diet Approach* (4th ed.), make the point that IE is a birthright. We were all born intuitive eaters. Think of a baby's or toddler's eating patterns. A baby will cry when he is hungry; he doesn't care that it hasn't been exactly three hours since the last time he ate. He is hungry *now* and will be telling his parents so until he is fed. When the baby is full, he stops eating. There is no forcing him to finish the meal. He clamps his mouth shut, turns his head away, and is distracted by everything else. He might play with his food or throw it to the dog. But to a baby, food is food and there are no morals yet. As we grew up in our diet culture, we learned to ignore our internal cues for hunger and fullness. We were taught to moralize food by labeling it "good" or "bad," and we were taught to moralize the sizes of our bodies.

There are ten IE principles set forth by Tribole and Resch. Remember that they are *principles*, not steps that have to be done in numerical order. The principles can be revisited as necessary in order to improve your intuitive eating skills. There is no finish line with IE. Everyone has their own relationship with food and body and therefore has their own intuitive eater strengths and weaknesses. Just in case you haven't read *Intuitive Eating* yet, I'm going to briefly explain each principle so that you can feel ready to go through the workbook and practice intuitive eating.

The Intuitive Eating Principles[47]

1. Reject the diet mentality.
2. Honor your hunger.
3. Make peace with food.
4. Challenge the food police.
5. Discover the satisfaction factor.
6. Feel your fullness.
7. Cope with your emotions with kindness.
8. Respect your body.
9. Movement—feel the difference.
10. Honor your health with gentle nutrition.

---

47 Tribole, Evelyn, and Elyse Resch. *Intuitive Eating: A Revolutionary Anti-Diet Approach.* 4th ed. New York: St. Martin's Press, 2020.

The first principle is the most important place to start: *reject the diet mentality*. This is how you will discern whether a program claiming to incorporate IE is actually a diet. By rejecting the diet mentality, you are saying that your dieting days are over. Striving for weight loss is also over. Those things do not serve your physical or mental health. As you start to practice IE, use this principle to check in with your thoughts and learn to catch yourself when the diet mentality sneaks in, as it does with Megan in the following example.

> Megan has been working on her IE skills for two months. She read the IE book and has been feeling hopeful about repairing her relationship with food. Megan also wants to be healthy and improve her cholesterol levels. She still feels that certain foods, such as chips or fast food, are not acceptable for her to eat because they will not help her cholesterol levels. Whenever she does eat these foods, she feels guilty for not nourishing her body the "right" way.

Megan has some work to do in rejecting a sneaky diet. That's the "wellness diet," a term created by fellow anti-diet dietitian Christy Harrison, creator of the podcast *Food Psych*. Although it is valid for Megan to want to improve her health, eating only for health reasons is actually a form of dieting, which often leads to stronger cravings for the forbidden foods. Eating does not need to be an all-or-nothing situation. Megan can improve her health and cholesterol levels, *and* still eat these foods when she has a craving.

Rejecting diet culture also involves ridding yourself of the things that promote dieting and the tools used to measure dieting success (or, in most cases, failure). The most obvious one is the bathroom scale. Weighing yourself should be restricted to specific circumstances, such as if you experience end-stage renal disease or congestive heart failure, when managing fluid accumulation is important. If the number on the scale is causing you guilt and turmoil, then it is time to get it out of the house. Other dieting tools may include the following:

- A food scale.
- A pedometer or exercise equipment (especially the equipment you never liked using anyway).
- Portion-control Tupperware.

- That goal swimsuit or clothing that you were planning to wear when you "lose the weight."

- A tape measure used to calculate waist or hip circumference.

- A scale or device that measures body composition, such as a bioelectrical impedance analysis device.

- Fitness apps, such as MyFitnessPal, Noom, Fooducate, Weight Watchers, SparkPeople, FatSecret, Fitbit, and so on.

- Weight loss recipe books or dieting books.

These tools served a purpose in your life at one point, but now you're going in a different direction. The faster they are purged from your house, the faster they can be off your brain. It's time to make room for the things that are going to bring you true happiness.

The *honor your hunger* principle sounds simple: eat when you are hungry. But this principle often trips people up. Chronic dieters have a long history of ignoring their hunger. Sometimes dieters don't ever feel hungry. This is part of the body's starvation-mode response. The body uses energy to release ghrelin, the hormone that makes you feel hungry. If these hunger cues are ignored for long enough, the body may decide they are not worth expending precious energy on anymore.

Think of it this way: your friend has been calling you, but you haven't felt like talking to her. You let the phone go to voicemail, and you ignore her texts. Eventually, she stops trying to communicate with you. One day you decide it would be nice to talk to this friend again, but when you call she lashes out at you. She wants to know what she did wrong for you to stop talking to her all of a sudden. You apologize, but will she forgive you or trust you again? Maybe. It will take a long time to regain her trust. It will take regular communication and consistently doing what you say you are going to do. Only then will your relationship start to get back to normal.

Your body is your friend. Through dieting, you ignored your friend's needs and she went on the offensive. You two fought nonstop. You wanted to look thinner, but she fought against your every effort. You start to realize that she was only protecting you. Even though you have stopped restricting food, she doesn't trust you yet. The two of you

56

need to rebuild what you broke down. She needs to trust that you are never going to do that again. Then you will both feel like friends again. When you are not fighting for control, she can be home.

To build back health and trust with your body, adequate nourishment is needed. This is one reason why working with a dietitian trained in intuitive eating is so important if hunger cues are missing or are quiet. A dietitian can provide individualized advice on how much and how often a new intuitive eater needs to eat in order to renourish their body. The hunger signals will eventually return.

Diet culture tries to demonize hunger and even presents methods to reduce appetite and therefore food intake. This separates you from your body's cues and creates chaos for your body systems. Feeling hungry is as normal as breathing or going to the bathroom. Eating is an essential task for life. There is nothing wrong with having a hearty appetite—in fact, it probably means you are healthy. There are different levels of hunger, which give you cues to what and how much you need to eat. Tribole and Resch advocate rating your hunger on a scale when first starting to pay attention to your hunger cues. Your scale might look something like this:

0: Not hungry at all. You are still full from the most recent time you ate.

3: A little hungry but not ready to eat something yet.

5: Hunger is more noticeable now. You're starting to think about food.

7: Definitely feeling hungry now. Your concentration is down and your stomach may be grumbling.

9: Feeling really hungry. Stomach is growling loudly. Your only focus is on eating right now.

10: Starving! Anything and everything edible sounds good right now. You may be irritable or grumpy.

Assess yourself right now using this scale. How hungry are you? When you've answered this question, decide what you're going to do with this information. Is it not yet time to eat? Is it time for a meal or snack? What do you need to do to honor your body's hunger level? Oftentimes we get busy and it is easy to ignore hunger cues. We may wait until we are a 9 or 10 on the scale and then feel out of control with food when we finally do eat. Or we might eat even if we are at 0 or 3, perhaps because we are bored. You may feel as though you eat all day long. Take these experiences as opportunities to grow and learn more about yourself. Think about what you can do differently next time to honor your hunger better.

It is normal for your hunger levels to fluctuate. You may feel more hungry on days when you have increased movement, such as when doing yard work, or during menstruation. Resist the diet mentality thoughts that might crop up on these days, such as, *I'm eating too much* or *I've eaten a lot today! No more until tomorrow.* Your food intake will balance out over time, with days when you don't feel as hungry. This is a much gentler and more natural process for your body compared with eating the same number of calories every day no matter what your hunger levels are. Start being mindful of your hunger throughout the day, and adjust your eating schedule to honor your hunger.

Many diets promote a set schedule for when a person can eat, such as every three to four hours. This tactic does not allow you to honor your hunger. You are an individual with a unique body. No single eating schedule is going to be right for every person. The same goes for fasting or intermittent fasting. When hunger signals are met with coffee or water instead of nourishing food, the body also processes this as starvation.

Make peace with food: recognize what moral value you place on foods. If you think, *I shouldn't eat that brownie. It's bad for me*, you have classified that food as "bad" or "unhealthy." If you think, *I've been so good today. I had a salad instead of choosing the pizza*, you associate eating salad with being "good" and pizza with being "bad." The goal of this principle is to erase these classifications.

Food is food. It is not good or bad. As I tell my clients, food does not make you automatically unhealthy or healthy. It is not fattening or slimming. Food can be neutral. For those who disagree, think about a person in your life who eats everything they want, no matter the food or the portion size, and is able to remain thin. Think of a person in your life (maybe you even) who eats the "cleanest" diet possible and remains heavier. People of all sizes and levels of "clean" diets still have health issues and disease.

When we strip away the moral context of food, we relieve ourselves of guilt, fear, anxieties, or shame about food. If eating pizza is not morally right or wrong, then there is no need to feel ashamed of eating it. If salad is chosen instead, it is because you thought that food sounded more appetizing in the moment. You are *giving yourself permission to eat all foods* and not allowing yourself to feel bad for eating what sounds good to eat.

The biggest benefit of making peace with food is halting the restrict-binge cycle. You know what this looks like: a certain food is off-limits because it is not on the diet plan or it is considered "unhealthy," but all you can do is think about that food. You crave it more than anything because it is forbidden. After much inner turmoil, you finally give in to the craving. You say it will be just one bite. That bite is so delicious, and you try to savor it. But it's gone before you know it, and you just gotta have more. That one bite turns into ten, and soon enough the whole thing is gone. And your craving still isn't satisfied. You're left feeling mad at yourself, ashamed of your "lack of self-control," as the diet industry puts it. You resolve to do better tomorrow. Maybe you try to set yourself up for success by keeping that food out of the house or avoiding social situations where you think it might be served. Thus you are back to restriction. As the cycle repeats itself, you are left feeling out of control with food.

Once you decide to make peace with food, no food is off-limits. This is the fun part, where you are allowed to break the rules. You don't feel guilty for eating anymore. Better yet, the cravings for certain foods diminish because you know you can have that food whenever you want. You have unconditional permission to eat.

This can feel scary. People worry that if they give themselves unconditional permission to eat, then they will eat huge amounts of those forbidden foods and feel even more out of control. They worry that they will gain weight or that they will feel hungry all the time and never stop eating. These fears are valid. Some people go through what is known as the honeymoon phase of intuitive eating. They do eat all the once-forbidden foods until they are finally satisfied. But then this phase ends. Their cravings diminish once the restriction is out of their systems. Now that you are building trust again with food and your body, you may need to prepare yourself to go through some challenging phases and big emotions. It is okay to go slowly. Consider the case of Macy.

Macy was grappling with the "make peace with food" principle of intuitive eating. She was terrified that if she gave herself permission to eat peanut butter, then she would eat the whole jar in one sitting. She loved peanut butter. She started by giving herself permission to eat other things previously restricted: cookies, fried chicken and mashed potatoes, and so on. When she ate these foods, she felt satisfied after eating them and told herself she could have more later if she wanted when she was hungry again. Only once or twice did she actually do this. Instead, she usually thought of something else that sounded better to eat.

Finally, she was ready to try incorporating peanut butter back into her life. It wasn't easy at first. Macy ate more than she wanted during her first trial. She felt guilty and somewhat sick to her stomach. She thought she had failed. She was reminded by her dietitian that she was allowed to eat however much she wanted. Any amount she chose to eat was okay. At the next trial, Macy tried practicing mindfulness while eating peanut butter. She tried to savor each spoonful and stopped eating a little sooner that time. She was pleased she didn't feel as sick. She told herself it was okay to stop now and have more later when she wanted more.

Macy took a little longer to make peace with peanut butter because of her past restriction-and-binge relationship with it. Ultimately, she was able to keep peanut butter in her house and even had some days when she didn't crave it at all. She felt great that it was no longer a trigger food. Once the restriction was removed and she trusted that she could eat it whenever she wanted, the bingeing ended. Remember, your body is the estranged friend who needs to rebuild trust with you, one bite at a time.

Challenge the food police is questioning the food rules or beliefs about your body that you have internalized. The food police voice tells you to follow diet rules and sends you on a guilt trip for breaking them. Setting an expectation or boundary with yourself and others is the first step to pushing back. Deciding on your boundaries is the easy part; putting them into practice and sticking to them is the hard part. Food policing is essentially shaming, although some people, like April's father in the next example, do it out of a desire to help.

April's father worried about his daughter's eating patterns. April asked for second helpings every evening at dinner. He didn't think a ten-year-old girl needed that much food, and most nights would tell her no. April watched with jealousy as her fourteen-year-old brother ate second and third helpings.

When they would go out to eat, April's father would criticize her menu pick and push her to get a salad instead. April would push back and the result was a meal ruined by everyone's sour mood. The older April got, the more comments she received from her father and eventually her friends. April stopped trusting herself with food because of comments such as, "Don't you think you should stop now? You've had a lot already" or "Are you really going to eat those cookies? If you're not hungry for an apple, then you shouldn't be eating at all."

The comments about her body were demeaning: "You would have a boyfriend if you just lost 15 pounds. You're getting fat. You need to eat less and exercise more." April tried dieting on and off for a year before she got serious about slimming her body. She started exercising for multiple hours every day and ate only three to four foods. As the pounds came off, she was praised and complimented. No one thought that she had an eating disorder.

Although her father thought he was helping, all April learned was that she could not trust her hunger cues. She thought her body was a problem, and the only solution was to create a thinner body. This led April to eating patterns that were disordered and hurt her mental health. April eventually found recovery in college but was still triggered by her father's comments when she visited home. Although it was difficult, she started setting boundaries with her father. She asked him not to make remarks about what or how much she was eating, or comment on her body. Her father didn't take this well, insisting that he was looking out for her and she was being too sensitive. Even though the conversation didn't go well, he thankfully did stop making these types of comments.

Not only do you need to set boundaries with others, but you also need to set them with yourself. Your inner food police is the strongest voice of them all. How many times have you beat yourself up for not looking a certain way or for eating the "wrong" foods? The unreasonable diet rules that you have followed are now being broken down by intuitive eating, and your inner food police may be rearing its ugly head.

In everyday eating situations, your inner food police will monitor your choices. You might recall that a certain diet said not to eat sooner than every three hours. The inner food police would convict you for eating your next meal early. Or you might remember that fruit has sugar and think about eating only half a banana even though you are hungry for a whole banana. Your inner food police says, *That was too much sugar! Do you want to get diabetes?!* Set the expectation with yourself that you will *not* let yourself believe those thoughts. Acknowledge them when they happen and actively forget about them.

It is time to turn off the policing voice and turn up the self-compassion voice. Would you say to your best friend that she was stupid or worthless for eating a cookie? If she had self-respect, she wouldn't be your friend for long. Remember, you are rekindling a friendship with yourself. Practice recognizing your negative self-talk, and enforce the boundary that you are no longer allowed to say those things to yourself. Negative self-talk causes feelings of hopelessness, fear, and despair. It's no wonder your behavior around food feels out of control.

It is time for your intuitive eater voice to be encouraged to speak up. Unlike dieting, intuitive eating has no rules. To start reconnecting with your body, meet yourself where you are. Let the self-compassion voice, or The Nurturer voice, as Tribole and Resch call it, bring out feelings of hope, calm, and positivity. You will start to discover self-awareness through being mindful.

Discover the satisfaction factor is all about choosing foods that please you. What do *you* like? What do *you* want to eat? Think about what flavors you like. Consider what food textures and temperatures are pleasing to your palate. If you are hungry, what food is going to hit the spot right now? Finding satisfaction in eating is the goal, but there are times when the satisfaction factor can be diminished. A few examples follow. Think of how you could change the situation (if possible) to allow your enjoyment of food to return.

- When you are invited out to dinner at your favorite restaurant, but you ate just twenty minutes earlier. Even eating your favorite meal is not as satisfactory when you are not hungry.

- When you haven't eaten all day and are ravenous. That meal will disappear so fast you won't even taste it.

- When you just had an argument. It's hard to enjoy your meal when you're in a bad mood.

- When your inner food police makes you feel guilty about what you chose to eat.

- When you eat only for health. The food you crave might not be the most nourishing food, and you might try eating other foods in an attempt to satisfy the craving. Ultimately, these foods won't satisfy you, so you might also eat the food you were craving anyway.

- When you are sick or your sense of smell is not great.

Making meals enjoyable is a large part of having a good relationship with food. Use your self-compassion voice and allow yourself to take pleasure in eating on all levels. I'm not talking about just taste. Find foods that satisfy a combination of your physical hunger, your tongue, your eyes, your nose (through smells), and even your emotional hunger.

I love meal variety. I don't want chicken for dinner or ice cream for dessert night after night. Experimenting with new food flavors, colors, and textures satisfies me on a deeper level. Choosing foods or food combinations that keep me full physically satisfies my body's hunger and allows me to have the energy and clear mind to do what is needed that day. Eating a variety of foods also supplies my body with a range of nutrients—but I'm getting ahead of myself here. Everyone will have a different eating style because we are all individuals. Your job is to find out what will be the most satisfying thing for you to eat in the moment. You don't have to always know what you want, but the more you practice tuning into what foods satisfy you, the better you will get to know your preferences.

Feel your fullness comes down to being mindful when eating. Many of us have learned that a person is "done" eating when the food is gone. You may have been a member of the "clean plate club" because you would be in trouble for wasting uneaten food. This method forces you to rely on external cues to stop eating. To feel your fullness, you must tune in to your internal sensations to determine when to conclude your meal. Practice mindfulness by rating your fullness level at various points in the meal and checking in with yourself on how the food is tasting.

0: Not full at all. You are still hungry.

3: A little full, but you're not ready to stop. The food is still tasting good.

5: Starting to feel full; you're starting to think about stopping soon.

7: Full. If you stop now, then you will feel satisfied and comfortable.

9: Too full! If you take another bite, then you might vomit. Food isn't tasting so good now.

10: So full you actually made yourself sick; you're incapacitated.

Although this sounds easy enough, many people struggle with this principle because they have not yet given themselves full permission to eat. Dieters who still fear restriction in type or amount of food cannot be expected to stop eating even when they are comfortably full. You may have heard of the "Last Supper" meal—a period of eating whatever you are craving, often in copious amounts, before starting the next diet. There is no eating in moderation when you will not be allowing yourself to eat these foods the next day. Even people who are not trying to diet for weight loss can have a last supper mindframe. I had a patient who was told that after his kidney transplant he could never eat raw meat again, so he constantly craved and ate sushi before his transplant to try to get his fill of it. Remember to give yourself permission to eat as much as you want, and keep in mind that you are allowed to have more later if you want it.

Many chronic dieters do not remember what it feels like to be comfortably full. They can't help but eat beyond a pleasant fullness level. This is Amy's story:

> Amy never seemed to feel full when eating. She always portioned out her food for fear that if she ate freely, then she might never stop. As a result, Amy felt hungry all the time. She even tried taking appetite suppressants at one point.

Amy wanted to become an intuitive eater but was struggling with the principle of "feel your fullness." Her dietitian told her these fears were normal and encouraged her to, just one time, try eating until she felt the need to stop. Amy's attempt to do so felt like a huge failure. She ate way more than she usually did and did not feel comfortably full. Instead, she felt sick. She had eaten past comfortable fullness without even noticing. When she told her dietitian, she was surprised to hear that was exactly what her dietitian had expected to happen. Her dietitian gave her new strategies to try on her next trial.

With this new information in mind, Amy tried again. She ate mindfully and without any distractions. As soon as she started to feel slightly sick, she stopped. The next time she ate, Amy remembered how much food she had eaten before feeling sick in her preceding trial, and she stopped before that point. And just like that, Amy wasn't hungry all the time. With practice, what once had felt out of control was now a guilt-free eating experience, and Amy knew she could trust her body to tell her when to stop eating.

When Amy put her attention on her target, that is, comfortable fullness, she was able to achieve it. Eating mindfully looks different for everyone, but typically it includes putting away distractions, such as your phone, book, or TV, and focusing instead on the experience of eating and what your body feels. Notice how the food smells before you take a bite. Assess how hungry you are. As you start to eat, think about the processes that your food went through to get onto the plate in front of you. Take a break when your plate is half eaten, put down your fork, and assess your fullness level. Assess your fullness level again when you decide you are done eating. All of this keeps you in tune with your body's sensations.

Remember that because you have given yourself unconditional permission to eat, you can respect your fullness and eat that same food again later if you still want it. No restriction means no rules. Have leftover spaghetti for breakfast if that sounds appetizing. You are in charge of deciding what food sounds good to eat, and how much is going to satisfy your appetite.

Because we are to find satisfaction and pleasure in food, this means that it is okay to eat food while feeling emotions (there is actually no way to eat while void of emotions). This takes us to the next principle, *cope with your emotions with kindness*. The "food is fuel" thinking does not account for the fact that in every culture, food accompanies celebrations, holidays, love, reward, and sometimes pain. In the United States, there are birthday cakes, Christmas dinners, and lollipops after getting a shot. A baby's crying is soothed with milk. A toddler is distracted with a cookie after a scraped knee. Food is therapeutic.

Emotional eating is something we all do, but it can look different for everyone. Some people eat when they are happy but have no appetite when they are upset or stressed. Others have a strong desire to eat when unpleasant feelings arise, such as stress, boredom, sadness, anger, or loneliness. In these instances, a person uses food to temporarily comfort themselves by distracting themselves from or numbing the unpleasant feelings. Preliminary research has found that a large risk factor for developing emotional eating is food restriction and dieting.[48, 49, 50] People who restrict food intake for weight control are more prone to emotional eating than intuitive eaters.

Emotional eating has been demonized by diet culture, which is ironic, because it appears that dieting is a main factor in why someone eats emotionally. It is seen as problematic and thought to contribute to why people gain weight. But emotional eating is an innocent act. Like someone who uses art to distract from difficult emotions, you may use food as a distraction. Emotional eating does not make you a bad person. The act of eating to cope has been lifesaving for you. There are certainly worse "substances" you could use to deal with the stress that life throws at you. Food is the easy, convenient coping option.

I used to advise my patients to refrain from emotional eating. I had no understanding of how emotional eating actually worked, and without intending to, I was just prescribing another diet. If my patient admitted to emotional eating, I would recommend they take

---

48 Amy T. Galloway, Claire V. Farrow, and Denise M. Martz, "Retrospective Reports of Child Feeding Practices, Current Eating Behaviors, and BMI in College Students," *Obesity* 18, no. 7 (2012): 1330–35, https://doi.org/10.1038/oby.2009.393.
49 Tracy L. Tylka, Julie C. Lumeng, and Ihuoma U. Eneli, "Maternal Intuitive Eating as a Moderator of the Association Between Concern About Child Weight and Restrictive Child Feeding," *Appetite* 95 (2015): 158–65, https://doi.org/10.1016/j.appet.2015.06.023.
50 Jordan Moy et al., "Dieting, Exercise, and Intuitive Eating Among Early Adolescents," *Eating Behaviors* 14 no. 4 (2013): 529–32, https://doi.org/10.1016/j.eatbeh.2013.06.014.

a bath, listen to music, go for a walk, or engage in some other stress-relieving activity instead of eating. The "instead" is why this was a diet. As soon as I told these people they could not use food to cope with stress, I was placing another food restriction on them. Just as with dieting for weight loss, when restriction was introduced, their cravings grew stronger, and they inevitably broke the rule and ate for emotional reasons. They were overcome with so much guilt that it erased whatever happiness they had just gained from emotional eating.

Instead of taking away your well-practiced coping mechanism of emotional eating, begin to *add* other coping skills to your playbook (you'll have a chance to explore this in Chapter 5). Principle number 3 still applies: you have unconditional permission to eat— yes, even when you are not physically hungry.

To cope with your emotions with kindness, you also need to meet your basic human needs. These include getting enough rest, expressing your feelings, feeling understood and heard, and receiving comfort. Even if you choose to continue emotional eating, this does not mean that you have failed at being an intuitive eater. You are choosing to support your mental health, which is just as important (if not more important!) than your physical health.

Focus on becoming the best intuitive eater you can be. As you become more attuned to your body's needs, you may find that your emotional eating gradually changes on its own. By honoring hunger and fullness, making peace with food, and nourishing the body adequately, the need to soothe with food can die down. After facing your feelings, they may not seem too big or scary to overcome with the other coping skills in your playbook. This is Chelsea's story:

> For Chelsea, food had been her coping method of choice since she was young. After a stressful day, TV and a bag of potato chips put her into a zoned-out state of mind, and she could forget all her problems—temporarily. When getting ready for bed, Chelsea would get mad at herself for eating all evening. She would say to herself, *If I didn't stress eat, then I wouldn't weigh so much! Tomorrow I'll be better. I'll work out instead of eat.*

Even if Chelsea did convince herself to go for a walk or do yoga after work, she still wound up stress eating to finally feel a release. To her dismay, she never felt peaceful at the end of the day because she always felt guilty for eating so much.

Chelsea decided to seek help from a professional to stop emotional eating. She started seeing a dietitian trained in intuitive eating and began her own intuitive eating journey. She started to recognize what feelings were leading her to emotionally eat and started seeing a therapist to help her process her stress and anxieties. Chelsea realized it felt better physically to not eat emotionally, which left her feeling heavy and bloated. She embraced the idea that she could still eat emotionally if she wanted to, and practiced releasing the mental restriction she was enforcing when she felt guilty for emotional eating.

Chelsea still eats emotionally sometimes but has found that she feels better physically when her emotional hunger is met through petting her cats or knitting while she watches TV at the end of the day. Her body size didn't change much even after she stopped eating emotionally daily. She is working through her feelings around internalized weight stigma and fatphobia with her therapist and dietitian to come to a place of body acceptance.

In this life you are given one body, which serves you in countless ways. *Respect your body* means something different to everyone, but taking care of your health is a great way to do this. That said, diet culture puts rules around bodies. Although you are trying to do what is best for your body, diet culture wants the opposite. By creating unattainable body size and shape standards, which sets the stage for self-hate and dissatisfaction, the diet industry can make money off your insecurities. No one who loves how they look and feel will buy diet supplements or diet programs, such as Slim-Fast or Weight Watchers.

I personally went through a long period of anger and grief about the diet industry because I felt tricked. I became a dietitian because I wanted to help people achieve health. I was taught that to do this, I needed to help them fix their body size. It is such a lie—a hidden one but obvious when you think about it. It is like saying that because I have blue eyes or brown hair that I am less healthy than someone who has green eyes or blonde hair. There are a million reasons why we look the way we do, including many things we have no control over, such as the culture we are raised in or our genetics. Diversity of body size is beautiful and does not mean that any one size is less healthy than another.

We do not truly respect our bodies if we are constantly trying to change them. I am at peace with my size 10 feet because I accept that they will never be small enough to fit into a size 8 shoe. Instead, I focus on the things I can control. If you are at war with your body, it will be difficult to fully make peace with food. You do not have to love, or even like, every part of your body, but you can still respect it for what it does for you. Tribole and Resch put it like this: "Respecting your body means treating it with dignity and meeting its basic needs." Your friend (that is, your body) needs kind words and positive affirmations, not condescending words or bullying. Has meanness ever helped anyone? If kind words do not come freely at first, start with neutrality. A belly is just a belly, a leg is a leg; that is a fact. Study the people in your life who make you feel loved and respected. Follow their example to talk to yourself in a loving and caring way.

You can respect your body with the final two principles (*movement—feel the difference* and *honor your health with gentle nutrition*), with the goal of overall health, not weight loss. I used to hate exercising because my goal was a flat stomach. Once my goal changed to having enough endurance and strength to do the things I wanted to do, my attitude toward exercise changed too. I found exercises that I liked, including walking, hiking, playing with my son and dog in the yard, and gardening. You see the common theme: I like to be outside. If you don't know what you like, experiment. You might discover a love for skiing or pickleball.

Most people have had bad experiences with exercise. One of my earliest exercise memories is having to run the mile in middle school PE. I remember thinking that I hated running. I actually love running, now that there are no rules about how long I have to run or how many calories I should burn. I can focus on how I feel when I move my body, which is much more important. I know I get better sleep after going for a hike, and my stress levels are lower.

Yoga, Tai Chi, Qigong, or similar practices are a great way to exercise with mindfulness. Yoga is usually gentle and soothing. Going slow and focusing on your breathing helps you connect with your body signals while you gain flexibility and strength. I always recommend yoga or chair yoga as a first step in getting back into movement again. A growing number of people are teaching and practicing yoga in a weight- and body-neutral way, which can support your path to body acceptance.

Moving your body in a way that feels good is being attuned to your body, but so is knowing when to rest. Diet culture pushes the idea that exercising three to five times per week, or even daily, is best for health. But this concept does not allow a person to take a day off if their body or mind doesn't feel like exercising, and can cause feelings of guilt. Listening to and honoring your body's need to rest is also practicing attunement. You do not need to feel guilty for following how you feel; no matter how many minutes per week of movement are recommended, no one knows your body as well as you do. By following your body's varying needs for movement *or* rest, you are respecting it.

Gentle nutrition puts into practice all the intuitive eating principles because you are honoring your health and your food cravings. It is the last principle discussed because this topic can trigger diet mentality thoughts and behaviors. The goal is to find a balanced way of eating that nourishes you, body and soul. Shush the inner food police pushing all-or-nothing thinking. The other principles still apply: you have permission to eat all foods in a way that satisfies you.

As an intuitive eater, you become mindful of how your body feels after eating certain foods. A stark example is food allergies. If you are allergic to peanuts, you know that if you eat them your body does *not* feel well afterward. For you, avoiding peanuts is eating intuitively. I remember as a kid I had a sudden craving for carrots after eating a lot of candy one day; I was in tune with what sounded good to my body. After I ate the carrots, I felt physically better.

Although a lot of research exists on which foods are the healthiest, try not to get lost in the weeds. Orthorexia, a condition characterized by an obsessive focus on eating healthy, can be just as bad as any other eating disorder. Your knowledge of nutrition can still serve you. If you are at the grocery store, picking out ground beef for taco night, you might be comparing the 85 percent lean meat with the 95 percent lean meat. Your inner nutrition expert might be saying, *Go for the 95 percent lean; it's healthier*, but your intuitive eater voice might be saying, *True, but that one just doesn't taste as good*. In this case, follow the intuitive eater voice and be more satisfied with your meal. If you think that they taste the same or the 95 percent lean meat tastes better, then choose the leaner meat. Stay flexible. Eat what sounds good and feels good in your body. If you need more guidance, your friendly intuitive eating dietitian is happy to help you support your nutrition.

I highly recommend that you read *Intuitive Eating: A Revolutionary Anti-Diet Approach* (4th ed.), whether now or later. Evelyn Tribole and Elyse Resch go into detail on each principle. Here are some IE research conclusions that support your decision to stop dieting and start eating intuitively:

- Intuitive eaters are 40 percent less likely to indulge in extreme weight control behaviors, and less likely to engage in chronic binge eating or dieting.[51]

- Intuitive eating is associated with significant improvements in psychological well-being indexes (for example, self-esteem, body appreciation, and optimism), cardio-metabolic parameters (blood pressure and cholesterol measures), and healthy behaviors (such as dietary and physical activity habits and nutritional quality of food).[52, 53, 54]

- Research shows that intuitive eaters do not tend to consume more high-fat or high-sugar foods than restrictive eaters. Intuitive eating is associated with a more varied and nutritious diet, as well as the adoption of healthy eating habits, such as eating breakfast.[55, 56, 57, 58]

These reasons, and the many others mentioned in this book, are why I urge people to give up dieting and intentional weight loss for good. A weight-inclusive approach works in achieving health and well-being, independent of weight loss. *There is no known way to safely and effectively induce significant and sustainable weight loss in the majority of people.* The Health at Every Size and intuitive eating approaches appear to be the only viable options in achieving real health.

---

51   Leslie Cadena-Schlam, and Gemma López-Guimerà, "Intuitive Eating: An Emerging Approach to Eating Behavior," *Nutrición Hospitalaria* 31, no. 3 (2014): 995–1002, https://doi.org/10.3305/nh.2015.31.3.7980.
52   Cadena-Schlam and López-Guimerà, "Intuitive Eating: An Emerging Approach."
53   Tylka et al., "The Weight-Inclusive Versus Weight-Normative Approach to Health: Evaluating the Evidence for Prioritizing Well-Being over Weight Loss," *Journal of Obesity* (2014), https://doi.org/10.1155/2014/983495.
54   Tribole and Resch, *Intuitive Eating*, 4th ed.
55   Cadena-Schlam and López-Guimerà, "Intuitive Eating: An Emerging Approach."
56   TeriSue Smith and Steven R. Hawks, "Intuitive Eating, Diet Composition, and the Meaning of Food in Healthy Weight Promotion," *American Journal of Health Education* 37, no. 3 (2006): 130–36, https://doi.org/10.1080/19325037.2006.10598892.
57   Bacon, Linda, and Lucy Aphramor, "Weight Science: Evaluating the Evidence for a Paradigm Shift," *Nutrition Journal* 10, no. 9 (2011): 69, https://doi.org/10.1186/1475-2891-10-9.
58   Tribole and Resch, *Intuitive Eating*, 4th ed.

Health at Every Size is becoming a popular movement as more people, including health care practitioners, realize that weight stigma and bias are major reasons why people stop eating intuitively and try to control their body size. HAES-based interventions have been shown to improve participants' diets, eating patterns, eating behaviors, anthropometric and metabolic parameters, as well as psychological well-being.[59] In embracing size diversity and letting go of the health and beauty ideals prominent in our culture, we adopt self-acceptance and self-respect.

Fat activists are speaking out in mainstream media about the harms of fatphobia, weight stigma, and diet culture. It's not surprising that they receive a great deal of pushback from people who still strongly believe fat is bad. Among the hate comments is another kind of comment: "I wish I could be as confident in my body as you are!" or "That's nice that you are okay with being that size, but I could never accept myself at that weight." But you *can* feel that way about your body too. HAES is not just for some people; it is meant for everyone.

Fat influencers became confident in their bodies because they rejected diet culture and found their body respect. Some even post pictures of themselves nude or in swimsuits or crop tops to normalize all body sizes and shapes and to show that health or beauty is not limited by weight or BMI. In the process of letting go of others' opinions, these men and women are reconnecting with themselves and discovering who they truly are.

This is a good time to acknowledge that throughout most of my life, I've lived in a thin body. I had thin-child privilege. I grew up never experiencing the many struggles and biases that people in larger bodies face. I moved through the world with relative ease, never questioning whether I took up too much space. But I was still affected by diet culture. I was fatphobic and, even though I was thin, I did not accept my body. I tell you this because thin privilege has allowed me the opportunities to be who I am and where I am today. But my voice is a supporting voice to all my fat allies. Their voices should be the loudest, but unfortunately, stigma often mutes their message. As you start to gain knowledge and confidence yourself, I hope you will share your perspective and experience with the world and support liberating people of size from discrimination.

---

59   Mariana Dimitrov Ulian et al., "Effects of a New Intervention Based on the Health at Every Size Approach for the Management of Obesity: The 'Health and Wellness in Obesity' Study," *Public Library of Science One* 13, no. 7 (2018), https://doi.org/10.1371/journal.pone.0198401.

The goal of this workbook is to help you live your happiest life, one in which you feel at home in your body, are satisfied with being you, know who you are, and love yourself as you are. This workbook utilizes journaling, mindfulness, and meditation to help you reconnect with your body, practice intuitive eating, and find food freedom. Being an intuitive eater involves being mindful of your physical sensations and emotional well-being. The prompts are intended to be completed journal style. But if meditation is more your speed, then most prompts can be reflected on instead.

Journaling provides a place for your thoughts. A journaling "brain dump" can even show you the intrusive beliefs you cling to. It serves as a record of your current feelings and emotions. You can look back at your writing and see the thoughts or beliefs that you want to let go of. You may decide to review your answers someday, and journal the same prompts again with your enhanced point of view and lived experiences.

There is no wrong way to do this. You can work through prompts and activities at your own pace. Some parts of the workbook might turn into habits you want to continue for the rest of your life. This is your opportunity to practice self-care and self-discovery. Everyone deserves time to work on themselves; no one can pour from an empty cup. Remember to practice self-compassion and forgiveness. Some parts of this workbook might trigger big feelings for you. Acknowledge this and allow yourself time and space to process them.

You might choose to go through this workbook at a time when life is a bit calmer. It may be difficult to truly dive into these topics when you are currently experiencing trauma or stress. If at any point in your journey you feel a desire to harm yourself, immediately tell a health care professional, such as your doctor or therapist. This book is not a substitute for individual medical or mental health advice.

Chapter 5

Anti-Diet Workbook

In this chapter, you will begin your guided practice of intuitive eating and find a happier relationship with food and your body.

Prompt

By recognizing which food rules you have integrated into your life, you will have the power to reject them and shush the inner food police. Food rules are restrictions made up by the diet industry. Some examples:

- Don't eat after 7:00 p.m.

- Sugar, carbs, fat, and so on are forbidden.

- Eat only X number of calories per day.

- Have protein shakes for breakfast and lunch daily.

- Fast on the weekends.

- You may have a cheat meal on Friday nights.

What are the food rules you have learned and practiced? Are there any food rules you apply to yourself currently?

....

....

....

....

....

....

....

Prompt

You and your body have been together for your whole life: through sickness and health, the good and the bad. Even if your current relationship with your body isn't great, you are making the choice to respect your body no matter what. No one can be expected to love, or even like, their body at all times, but we can learn to shift away from negativity to neutrality and positivity out of respect.

How do you see your body right now? Make a list of adjectives to describe how you perceive your body, such as short or tall, strong or frail, or elegant or awkward.

....

....

....

....

....

....

....

How does this compare with how you think others see you? Does the way others perceive your body matter to you right now, and why or why not?

....

....

....

....

....

....

....

WHY DO I EAT? ACTIVITY

Intuitive eating involves paying attention to why you start and why you stop eating. The following examples are factors affecting why someone chooses to start eating, stop eating, or not eat at all:

Start Eating

- Feeling physically hungry (stomach growling, thinking more about food, lack of concentration, headache, and so on).

- Emotional eating (emotions could be either positive or negative).

- Boredom.

- Someone offers you a snack that you eat so as not to appear rude.

- Your next opportunity to eat won't be for several hours (e.g., eating something before work).

- Everyone else around you is eating.

- You are in a specific location or situation, such as at the movie theater, where everyone is eating popcorn.

Stop Eating

- Feeling physically full (food doesn't taste as good; feeling content and satisfied).

- The food is gone or the plate is clean.

- Feeling sick or overstuffed.

- You get distracted, such as when you take a phone call.

- The allotted time to eat has ended, such as the end of a work break.

Choose Not to Eat

- Feeling physically full (nothing sounds good to eat; still full from last meal or snack).

- The food offered doesn't look appetizing or is something you dislike or are allergic to.

- Emotional reasons, for example, you are anxious or depressed.

For the next twenty-four to forty-eight hours, tune into what factors you use to decide when to start eating, stop eating, or choose not to eat. Make a list of these observations for each category.

Prompt

An intuitive eater stops to think about what sounds good to eat when they are feeling hungry. They have to determine what they are hungry for in the moment. When you have unconditional permission to eat all foods, sometimes cravings are not as pronounced compared with your dieting days, when cravings were obvious and strong.

What foods are you craving today? What kinds of foods did you crave in the past during your dieting days? For the next three days, keep a running list of the foods you crave.

Day 1	Day 2	Day 3

Prompt

Although there are objective definitions of health, we all have a subjective opinion on what health means to us. What does healthy look like for you in your body? How has that definition changed over time? What do you feel influences your thoughts about what is healthy versus unhealthy?

....

....

....

....

....

....

....

Prompt

When I was growing up, someone in my family was always on a diet. I watched them avoid the desserts at family gatherings and overheard them talking about how much weight they were trying to lose. That influenced how I thought about people in bigger bodies—that they were not healthy, that they were not beautiful, and that they were not normal. Although I had the privilege of growing up in a thin body, I felt the need to watch my body and be careful that I never gained too much weight. I was worried fatness was in my genetic makeup, so I thought I needed to be mindful to eat the "right" foods and exercise enough to prevent it from happening to me. I thought being fat was a terrible thing because that was what everyone made it out to be. (This was even more true when I started working in health care.)

Think about your own experiences with diet culture growing up and as an adult. How did these experiences shape your thoughts about bigger bodies and your own body? What kinds of words or descriptors do you associate with being fat?

FINDING JOY IN EATING ACTIVITY

A diet mentality (or even a health-focused mentality) can cause you to have a love–hate relationship with food. For example, you may eat a doughnut because you crave it but then worry it will add an inch to your waistline or somehow ruin your health with one helping! Guilt sucks all the enjoyment and fun out of eating. Or maybe you've tried meal prepping for the coming week in order to "be good" and avoid eating out, only to experience the boredom of eating the same meal again and again.

Now that you are giving yourself unconditional permission to eat what and when you desire, you can rekindle the joy in eating. By being intuitive (and through a little trial and error), you will discover what foods sound good to you and when food will be the most tasty and enjoyable. Your hunger level factors into this. You want to find a sweet spot, not so ravenous that you can't taste the food as you finally eat it, and not so satiated that nothing sounds or tastes all that good. Our bodies are intelligent and will tell us what they need in the moment.

Using your developing skills of self-awareness, rate your hunger level three times throughout the day today. Based on each rating, decide if you want to eat at that moment or wait a little longer. When you are ready to eat, ask yourself these questions:

1. Am I hungry for a meal or a snack?

2. Out of any food in the world, what do I *want* to eat? (Revisit your cravings prompt (see page 79); consider what you have time to purchase or prepare.)

3. How can I make my eating experience even more enjoyable? Sitting outside (or at least away from the desk)? Putting down a nice tablecloth?

Think about what aspects of eating your food would make it the most pleasurable, and implement your ideas.

RAISIN ACTIVITY

There are many different versions of this mindful eating activity online. If you would rather listen to this activity, several audio recording options will walk you through it. For this activity, put away any distractions and find a place where you can concentrate for a few minutes. To begin, obtain a raisin or another food of your choosing. (I highly recommend something sweet, such as an M&M or a graham cracker.)

1. Place the raisin on the table or plate before you.

2. Notice everything about the way it looks: the color, the wrinkles, and so on. Does it look as though it will be hard or soft when you bite into it?

3. Think about the process it went through to sit in front of you today. Maybe it started as a grape in a California vineyard. It was planted, watered, and tended. Then it was picked, dehydrated, packaged, and shipped to your local grocery store, where you purchased it and brought it home. Take a moment to be grateful for this process.

4. Pick it up and notice how it feels in your hand. Roll it around in your palm. Squish it between your fingers.

5. Notice its smell. Did your mouth start to salivate at the smell, or when you thought about eating it?

6. Place it in your mouth without chewing it. Let your tongue roll it around in your mouth. Do you taste anything? Notice the texture again.

7. Let yourself chew and fully taste it. Enjoy the flavor and sweetness. Did your tongue automatically put it to one side of your mouth?

8. As you start to swallow, notice how your tongue knows exactly how to move. Feel the food move down into your esophagus. Hold onto how the raisin tasted for a second more.

The activity is that simple. Repeat as often as you'd like or with different foods to practice eating mindfully. This practice creates a stronger connection to your body through self-awareness of your senses.

Prompt

You have devoted so much time, energy, thought, and more into changing your body. By giving up dieting, you free yourself up for so much! What things make you happy? List as many things as you can, thinking about all areas of your life. How can you set yourself up to do at least one of these things this week?

FEELINGS AND FOOD JOURNAL

We all eat emotionally to some extent. The first step in deciding you want to change how you cope with negative feelings is to be aware you are feeling them. For the next three days, document your day-to-day feelings and the reasons for them in detail. You can journal how you chose to cope and how you felt afterward.

Example

Feeling	Why?	How did I cope?	Do I feel better?
Stressed	A customer gave me a really hard time with...	I ate chips.	Yes & no because...

The point of this journal is to be attuned to your feelings and know why you are needing to cope through eating when you are not biologically hungry. Remember, it is okay to eat emotionally because you have unconditional permission to eat! It is a coping mechanism, just like reading or going for a walk.

Feeling	Why?	How did I cope?	Do I feel better?

EATING WITHOUT DISTRACTION ACTIVITY

Many people multitask when eating. They watch TV, work, or play a game on their phone. But this distracts the mind from how the body feels during food consumption. More often than not, the end of the meal comes when the food is gone, or when you start to feel ill from eating from eating past comfortable fullness.

For the next twenty-four hours (or longer) challenge yourself to eat with as little distraction as possible. Pay attention to how your food tastes and how your body feels when eating. Feel your fullness and enjoy your meal. If there are occasions when you must eat and do other things at the same time, be aware that you are choosing to eat while distracted, and notice if your eating experience is as enjoyable or satisfying.

Prompt

Make a list of foods that were "off-limits" for you in your dieting days. Write down specific foods versus general terms, such as *sweets*, and even narrow it down to the brand names if you can. Think about foods that feel scary to you or that you avoid because you believe they cause weight gain or hurt your health in some way. Also add foods to this list that you worry will trigger a binge episode. Consider all flavor profiles, such as salty, sweet, spicy, sour, savory, bitter, umami, and so on. As you remember more foods, add them to this list.

PLEASE THE EYES ACTIVITY

Many times our eyes are looking to enjoy food just as much as our tongues are. I once walked into a coffee shop for some much-needed caffeine and saw an assortment of cookies in the display case. Normally, sugar cookies aren't my sweet of choice, but these ones had beautiful designs in the icing, such as little hearts, and some had colorful sprinkles. My eyes were pleased by those cookies, and my mouth watered, wanting to taste one. Combined with the ambience of the shop and my black coffee, it was a memorable treat.

In this activity, you are going to create your own beautiful and enjoyable atmosphere to eat in. This practice will help you find joy and satisfaction in eating by satisfying your eye hunger. There are many factors to consider in making your meal beautiful. You can make your eating space as simple or extravagant as you'd like. Consider doing the following as you create your personalized beautiful eating environment:

- Choose whether to eat inside or outside.

- Clean off the table; add a nice tablecloth or place mats.

- Choose tableware that is visually pleasing; even consider your salt and pepper shakers, napkins, and butter dish.

- Arrange your food on the plate as beautifully as it would be at a restaurant; play with adding different colors or textures to your plate.

- Add a garnish, such as a parsley sprig, chopped green onion, a lemon wedge, or edible flowers.

- Light a candle and dim the lights.

- Add flowers or another centerpiece to your table.

- Put on music that makes you feel peaceful; have fun making your own playlist.

- Put away distractions, such as your phone, so you can fully take in your surroundings.

- If you feel like it, you can even dress up to match the environment.

Take a moment to appreciate the atmosphere you created, and then enjoy your meal. At the end of the meal, feel free to linger for a few minutes and soak up the satisfaction.

Prompt

Think about what you say when you talk to yourself, whether silently or out loud. You are the person you talk to the most. What are you thinking when you look at yourself in the mirror, or as you go about your day? Write down this inner monologue today.

REFRAMING SELF-TALK ACTIVITY

To respect your body, you must treat it with dignity. That includes talking to yourself the way you would a friend. Negative self-talk rarely motivates anyone. It mostly just hurts. An important thing to acknowledge is that at some point in your life, someone showed you how to talk to yourself like this. No one is born disliking themself.

In this activity, you will challenge your beliefs about yourself. You must decide if the thought you are having is intrusive and if you will reject it. You are always able to reframe a thought in a more positive light.

Continue to practice being aware of how you talk to yourself (refer back to your inner monologue journal entry on page 88). When you catch yourself participating in negative self-talk, practice reframing the thought into something respectful, positive, or even loving.

Examples

Negative Self-Talk	Reframed Sentence
I can't believe I was so dumb. I forgot to put my gym bag in the car.	I accidently forgot my gym bag. Oh well, everyone makes mistakes. It's such a nice day, I can go for a walk later instead if I feel like it.
I'm so bad for eating that cupcake at work.	I really enjoyed that cupcake, and I felt that I connected with everyone else in the moment instead of leaving the room like I would have in the past. I do not need to feel guilty for eating a cupcake.
My body is not good enough to wear a swimsuit.	Why am I worried about what others think of me? I think my body looks hot in this swimsuit, and I'm going to wear it because I like it!
I don't look as good in this dress as the model did online.	I shouldn't compare myself with others. This dress fits my body differently from the model's because we have different bodies. I am allowed to feel beautiful in my current body. The only person I want to impress is me.

Can you see that in the reframed sentences there is self-compassion, self-love, and even self-forgiveness? If you are struggling to reframe a thought, try using a positive affirmation that starts with "I am _____" (for example, "I am smart," "I am beautiful," or "I am determined").

If this is a big jump from the way you speak to yourself now, try taking a neutral approach. Decide if the negative thought is a fact or your opinion. Although facts can't change, opinions can. You have the power to change your opinions. In reframing negative thoughts as neutral thoughts, start by stating just the facts.

Examples

Negative Self-Talk	Stating the Facts
I can't believe I was so dumb. I forgot to put my gym bag in the car.	I forgot to put my gym bag in the car today. Next time I can set a reminder on my phone to help me remember.
I'm so bad for eating that cupcake at work.	Eating a cupcake does not make me a bad person. The fact is, eating a less-nutritious food is not going to make me instantly unhealthy.
My body is not good enough to wear a swimsuit.	My body is good, no matter how I look. The only opinion that matters is mine. I choose to swim in something more comfortable than a baggy T-shirt and shorts.
I don't look as good in this dress as the model did online.	This is not a fact but my opinion, which I have the power to change: she looks beautiful in this dress and so do I.

Write down your reframed thoughts as a reminder. Observe how in time it gets easier to reframe your thinking.

....

....

....

BODY GRATITUDE AND PROGRESSIVE MUSCLE RELAXATION ACTIVITY

Many versions of this activity have also been created, as well as audio versions. Read all the steps first and then try this out.

Sit or lie down in a comfortable position. Close your eyes and focus your attention on your breath. Relax for a minute or two. If your mind wanders away from your breath, that's okay. Just come back to noticing your breath again.

Next, think about your toes. Contract them as hard as you can, and hold that contraction for three seconds. Relax your toes completely and feel the sensations. Think about how your toes serve you and thank them: "Thank you, toes, for keeping me balanced when I stand and walk."

Think about the rest of your feet: the balls of your feet, the tops of your feet, your heels, and your ankles. Point your feet and hold the contraction for three seconds before relaxing. Think about how your feet serve you and thank them: "Thank you, feet, for carrying me where I need to go in the world."

Notice your legs: your calves, shins, knees, and thighs. Contract each muscle as hard as you can for three seconds. Then relax. Think about all the ways your legs serve you and thank them: "Thank you, legs, for standing, walking, running, jumping, skipping, dancing, and climbing."

Notice your belly and how it rises and falls when you breathe. Contract your abdominal muscles for three seconds and then relax completely. Reflect on how your belly serves you and thank it: "Thank you, belly, for housing the organs that digest my food and clean my blood."

Notice your chest and how it also rises and falls when you breathe. Round your shoulders in and contract your chest muscles for three seconds. Relax these muscles. Thank your chest: "Thank you, chest, for housing my heart and lungs, organs I could not live without."

THE **ANTI-DIET** WORKBOOK

Notice your glutes, back muscles, and shoulder muscles resting against the chair or bed. Contract all the muscles in these areas for three seconds before relaxing them. Consider how they serve you and thank them: "Thank you, strong back, for keeping me upright, and for being able to move, bend, and twist in the directions I need."

Notice your arms: your upper arms, elbows, and lower arms. Contract these muscles for three seconds. Relax them and thank them for how they serve you. "Thank you, arms, for carrying and reaching for the things I need—and for giving hugs and cuddles."

Notice your hands and fingers. Make fists and contract your hands for three seconds. Relax your hands and focus on relaxing each finger. Thank your hands and fingers for how they serve you: "Thank you, hands and fingers, for holding, opening, writing, typing, sharing, feeding, bathing, creating, and so much more."

Notice your neck and head. Contract your neck muscles for three seconds, and then relax them. Thank your neck and head for how they serve you: "Thank you, neck, for holding up my head. Thank you, head, for housing my smart brain."

Notice your face. Scrunch up your face and hold the contraction for three seconds. Relax your face, tongue, and jaw. Thank each part of your face for how it serves you. "Thank you, mouth, for tasting, chewing, and enjoying food. Thank you, nose, for the sweet smells you have given me, which bring back memories. Thank you, ears, for hearing words and music. Thank you, eyes, for beholding my world."

As you close this activity, bring your mind back to your breath, and relax in this position for as long as you'd like.

FINDING SATISFACTION IN EATING ACTIVITY

This activity is similar to the Finding Joy in Eating activity on page 82, but instead of focusing on hunger levels, you will be focusing on your fullness. Remember the 0 to 10 fullness scale in Chapter 4. You'll likely find that meal satisfaction is highest when you eat until you are comfortably full. Eating too little food can leave you looking to eat more, and eating too much food can leave you feeling sick or uncomfortable.

Finding satisfaction also comes from enjoying what you are eating. Do you think if you ate the same thing for dinner every day you would find joy in eating it and satisfaction when you were done? Or would you be looking for something else to eat ten minutes later? Most people desire a variety of foods to satisfy their palate.

You may find that sometimes food won't satisfy you in the way you thought it would. I remember once going to my in-law's house to celebrate my son's birthday. His Gigi made a wonderful dinosaur cake from scratch, and I was so excited to taste it! When it was finally time, the lemon-flavored cake was dished up and I tried a bite. In that moment, I admit I was disappointed. Although it tasted nice and sweet, I realized it just wasn't what I wanted. I was still full from a yummy lunch an hour earlier, and my stomach and taste buds were not interested yet in that cake. In the past I may have eaten it anyways or taken a piece home even though it wasn't my favorite. This time, I followed my body's intuitive cues and left most of the cake uneaten on the plate. I suspect I may have hurt Gigi's feelings, but it was more important for me to listen to my body. I would not have enjoyed the rest of our visit if I were feeling sick and overstuffed.

For the next twenty-four hours (or longer), practice finding satisfaction in eating. In doing so, consider the following:

Ask yourself what you feel like eating right now.

Eat in a mindful way as you have practiced, with limited distractions.

When your plate is halfway eaten, put your fork down and consider where you are on the fullness scale. Rate yourself and determine if you are going to continue eating. Will the food still taste good if you keep eating? If you stop now, will you feel satisfied with the meal? If you decide to keep eating, check in again with yourself later.

After you have decided to stop eating, ask yourself, *Do I feel satisfied or do I need something else?* If you decide you need something else, think about what you are craving in that moment and satisfy your craving.

FOOD CHALLENGE ACTIVITY

This activity is one of the hardest ones for some people. It's okay to feel anxious or nervous. There is a lot of brain rewiring to do, and an entire diet culture to unlearn. You are in the process of rebuilding trust with your body, and this activity is a big trust fall. You are proving to yourself that your body knows what you need and that you can trust yourself to eat anything in any amount, and still be okay. You are proving that you can show yourself respect, no matter what happens with food. It may be good to choose low-stress days to complete this challenge.

By now you have created a list of foods that were previously deemed "off-limits" or triggering foods from your dieting days. Starting with one that is likely the least triggering for you, select a food for your first food challenge. You may choose to rank the foods on your list for the purpose of this activity.

You will be eating this food (and all of them eventually) using your intuitive and mindful eating skills. Before you start, remember this: in order to avoid self-induced guilt, you must give yourself unconditional permission to eat all foods at the times and in the amounts that satisfy you. Whatever happens, this is an experiment that will give you information that you can work with.

Once you've selected your food, it's time to go get it. Make sure to purchase or make enough. You may want to purchase or make more than enough if you are triggered when you feel you can't get enough of this food or have limited opportunities to eat this food. If you have an abundance, you will know that you still have more opportunities to eat it again later and not fall into the "Last Supper" mentality. Remember, you can always have more later if that food still sounds good.

When you've put away any distractions and you've got your food in front of you, take a few deep breaths. Start your intuitive and mindful eating process:

- Rate your hunger level.

- Think about how your food is going to taste.

- Is the smell of it making your mouth water?

- Does it look the way you remembered it? Notice the color, texture, and temperature as you get ready to take your first bite.

- Take your first bite and chew it slowly. Put your utensil down and close your eyes; notice all the flavors flooding your mouth.

- After you have swallowed, take your next bite. Rate how much you enjoy this food on a scale of 0 to 10.

- Continue to eat this food mindfully and take a break when your plate is half eaten.

- Rate your fullness level.

- Rate your satisfaction level from 0 to 10. Does the food still taste as good as those first few bites?

- Decide if you would like to keep eating. Remember the circumstances of all the times you felt the most satisfied after eating. And remember your self-compassion if you eat past comfortable fullness this time; you're gathering information.

After you have finished eating, note your final fullness level and satisfaction level. If your inner food police voice is coming out, tell that voice to shush. You are allowed to feel happy and satisfied after eating anything you want in any amount you want.

Ask yourself this final question: Did that food taste as good as you had remembered? If so, this is a food you may want to incorporate into your regular food rotation. You can eat it as often as you like. If it didn't taste as good as you remembered, decide if you are going to try it again at a later date, or forget about it for a while and move on to finding foods that satisfy you more.

Continue to challenge all the foods on your list in this way until there is not one food that is still off-limits to you. You may choose to work with a support person or a registered dietitian or therapist with experience in conducting food challenges. Remember to extend compassion and forgiveness to yourself for your old ways and habits. Body trust and food freedom are coming into full swing!

INTUITIVE SHOPPING ACTIVITY

There was a time when I would plan out everything I would eat, every meal and every snack. I usually planned a week in advance and then based my shopping list off my meal plan. I bought only what was on the list in an attempt to keep "junk" out of the house, so I couldn't consume it all in one night. All my good intentions usually were out the window by day two. The snacks I had planned were not what I was craving. The meals I had planned no longer sounded good. I would open every cabinet and drawer, looking for something to eat that matched what I was craving. Most times I was left feeling unsatisfied to the point where I would go and buy fast food or candy just to curb that craving.

Do you identify with my experience with meal planning? Making a shopping list or planning out meals for the week can be a necessary and practical task. If you like to be organized like that, who am I to stop you? But the key is flexibility. Plans change, energy levels wax and wane, or you change your mind on what sounds satisfying to eat. Allow yourself flexibility and freedom to stray from the plan.

Sometimes having a plan for what to eat helps you honor your hunger. Waiting too long to decide what to eat can put you too high on the hunger scale. Then you're hangry (hungry *and* angry). When creating a meal plan or shopping list, get a sense of what sounds good to eat currently. You may even want to look up pictures of food on Google Images or Pinterest to spark your interests. If following the meal plan works out, that's great. If not, stay flexible.

Then, the next time you are in the grocery store, get the items from your list, and also see if any other foods speak to you. Roam every aisle to see what else looks good. For example, you might see a can of diced pineapple and remember a super yummy baked ham recipe with a brown sugar, clove, and pineapple glaze! You can gather ingredients for that recipe too and know that meal will be enjoyable and satisfying. I call this intuitive shopping. Let your taste buds do the shopping and your food freedom flourish!

Prompt

Although you might not love every part of your body, you can treat it with honor and respect. There are so many amazing things your body does that you might forget about! It can heal itself, from the smallest scrapes to broken bones. The heart beats and the lungs breathe all on their own. It sends you signals that it needs to eat or go to the bathroom. Anyone who has experienced any fault in body processes through illness has another level of appreciation when the body is working properly again. Take a moment to think about all the amazing things your body can do. What is a part of your body that you are grateful for today? What is a part of your body that you like today?

EMOTIONAL EATING ACTIVITY

When you find yourself eating for reasons beyond physical hunger, ask yourself why. Just as with becoming attuned to your hunger and fullness cues, you can become attuned to and curious about what you are feeling (think back to your feelings journal entries on page 85). If you have the goal of lessening occurrences of emotional eating, then first make sure you are not restricting food (physically or mentally). Then, instead of replacing your eating coping skill, add other possibilities to your playbook. When you are deciding how to accomplish what you need, you can choose the right coping option for the job.

There are many different categories of coping skills to consider. Some of the examples that follow could belong to more than one category. Take a minute to review these coping skills and add your own to the list.

Comfort and Relaxation

When you determine you need something that brings you good memories and feelings of gentleness, pleasure, or peace, try one of these activities:

- Go for a leisurely walk.

- Pull on a cozy blanket (or try a weighted blanket).

- Start a fire in the fireplace, and grab a cup of tea or cocoa.

- Sit outside and listen to nature or the rain. (There are apps that let you listen to nature sounds, birds, rain, ocean waves, and so on.)

- Snuggle or play with your pets.

- Put on your favorite happy music.

- Lie in a hammock.

- Get a manicure/pedicure, facial, or massage.

- Amuse yourself with Play-Doh, slime, or kinetic sand.

- Sit in a sauna or hot tub.

- Watch the sunset or sunrise.

- Swing on a swing.

- Bring in fresh flowers.

- Do yoga or chair yoga.

- Walk outside barefoot.

- Practice deep breathing exercises.

- Sing or dance.

- Sit in the sun (don't forget your SPF).

Distract and Dull

It is okay to take breaks from your feelings! Try these activities when you determine you need to zone out:

- Read an attention-grabbing book.

- Play a mindless game on your phone or computer.

- Watch a movie or TV show; go to the movies.

- Work on a jigsaw puzzle, crossword puzzle, word search, sudoku, and so on.

- Knit, crochet, embroider, sew, or quilt.

- Draw, color, or paint.

- Scrapbook.

- Garden or try a Zen garden.

- Play an instrument.

- Try photography.

- Scroll social media (just beware of people who promote diet culture).

- Take a nap.

- Play a board game or card game.

- Clean and organize.

- Play with a bead stress ball, a Push Pop Bubble Fidget Sensory Toy (from RadBizz), or other anxiety-reducing toys.

Feel the Feelings

Sometimes the best way to move past a negative emotion is just to feel it. This can be difficult, scary, and uncomfortable. We don't like feeling unpleasant things, and the body's natural reaction is to get away from or stop them! But pushed-down emotions crop back up eventually. At times, addressing them head-on is the best course of action:

- Journal about how you're feeling (you could write it down or even record a video).

- Meditate; sit with the feelings while taking deep breaths.

- Take a drive to think.

- Talk to a trusted person about your feelings.

- Release your emotions with a good cry. Watch a sad movie or put on sad music to help bring on the tears.

- Beat up a punching bag or pillow if physical energy needs to be released.

- Confront the offender.

In this activity, pick out a few coping skills from the preceding lists. When you feel yourself reaching for food but sense you are not physically hungry, take a short time out and ask yourself the following:

What emotions am I feeling right now?

What do I need at this moment to feel better?

What will help me accomplish this in the best possible way?

For example: *I am feeling rejected and mad because my friend canceled our plans at the last minute to hang out with her boyfriend instead. I need to forget about what happened for a while. I don't want to deal with these feelings right now. I can accomplish this by eating and watching TV, or I can lose myself in that book that kept me up way too late last night. I think I'll start with the book, and if I still feel like eating after ten minutes or so, I can.*

If a coping skill other than eating will meet your needs, you can decide to choose it. There may be times when your emotions are too big to consider anything but eating to cope with them. That is okay! Instead of feeling guilt, practice being grateful that you have a way to cope with something so big. Work on incorporating more coping skills into your life that match what you need in the moment.

Important Note

Although emotional eating can be an innocent coping skill, it is harmful when it causes large interferences in a person's life. Binge eating is a prime example of this. When people binge, they feel out of control with food, like they are treading water in the deep end of the pool with no way out. You deserve to feel comfortable in your body, not overstuffed or sick from eating (some call this overeating). When emotional eating becomes a secret or makes you physically ill, it may be time to work with an experienced intuitive eating dietitian or Health at Every Size–aligned therapist, who can help guide you back to the shallow end of the pool.

Prompt

As I became an intuitive eater and a person who was trying to reject diet culture, I had a lot of feelings about my weight and size. I truly believed intuitive eating was my destiny, but I still had one foot in diet mentality territory because I continued to hope I could lose weight someday. Even understanding all the risks that come with dieting and trying to intentionally change body size or weight, I still thought that somehow it would be possible for me. Eventually, I realized I was trying to process my new reality and was actually grieving. I was grieving the thought that I might not ever have a smaller body. That I might never fit into a size 8 again. That I might always carry more weight around my middle.

The grief then morphed into anger. I hated that I had been tricked into thinking that I would feel accepted or beautiful only in a smaller body. I hated that Western society was taught to think that way. Most of all, I hated that my son, and many other young people, were currently growing up to think this too. The anger is still strong some days, but it is also morphing into something else: acceptance. Without acceptance of my own body, I would never have been able to try to help someone else accept their body. Without accepting my body, I could never show my son, my brother and sisters, or my niece what it means to live a full life in a larger body.

Not all days are body-positive days. Some days I have intrusive thoughts that make me consider trying to change my body. I think my acceptance of my body is not going to be a linear process. I strive for progress, never perfection. I will press on in treating my body with respect. Someday I will embody the change I want to see in others.

What does it look like for you to let go of the dream of weight loss? What do you have to grieve or mourn? What are you angry about? What are the positive things you will gain from renouncing this goal?

....

....

....

....

....

....

....

....

Prompt

When the only thing you focus on is your body or your weight, all other aspects of life can get neglected. But you have only one lifetime. It's time to decide that your body is the least interesting thing about you. It's time to stop caring about the opinions of others. It's time to finally focus on what makes you happy. What are the desires you have for your life? Consider where you want to be and what you want to be doing in the next five or more years regardless of your size. Now zoom in on today. Set one to three goals or tasks you want to accomplish today. Get your mind off your looks, and focus on what really matters in life.

....

....

....

....

....

....

....

....

Prompt

I've heard many different reasons for why someone wants to lose weight, but by far the most common one is, "I'll feel more comfortable in my body after I lose weight."

Diet culture wants us to believe that weight loss is the best way—indeed, the only way—to feel more comfortable. Fat people have a different set of physical issues when it comes to their bodies. You may be challenged by one or more of the following:

- Feeling uncomfortable in clothes that once fit you—but no longer.

- Struggling to find clothing in your size, let alone clothes that are reasonably priced and stylish.

- Hygiene.

- Skin irritation; cracks in skin folds.

- Excessive sweat and heat under breasts or in skin folds.

- Chafing thighs.

- Feeling out of breath with minimal exertion.

- Inflexibility.

- Limited strength or endurance.

But all these complaints have solutions that do not involve losing weight. Seriously, a quick Google search pulls up all kinds of good resources. A great one I've found is the website comfyfat.com. The founder, J. Aprileo, provides clothing and product suggestions for fat people. Clothing stores are starting to listen to the criticisms of plus-size fashion (although they have a long way to go). You can find consumer reviews and clothing haul try-ons all over social media these days. To feel more comfortable in your clothes, start by wearing clothes that fit. Find clothes that you like wearing and feel beautiful in.

Nowadays many products are available to improve hygiene and prevent skin breakdown in areas that rub or are hard to keep dry. For example, a detachable shower head and a long-handled loofah are must-have shower accessories for feeling your cleanest. There are bra or tummy liners and spray or roll-on deodorants that can be used on potentially sweaty days. Consider using an attachable bidet on your toilet if reaching behind to wipe yourself clean is troublesome. A world of answers is out there.

There are talented fat athletes, personal trainers, yoga instructors, runners, and gymnasts who prove to the world that fat bodies can be strong and flexible too. If you want to get out of a chair or tie your shoes more easily, you can train for it! If you want to prevent disability or the need for a caretaker later in life (which many thin people require too, by the way), you don't need to lose weight! Instead, you must build a strong body that can keep up with what you want to do. There are helpful assistive devices out there too, such as the Sock On/Sock Off kit or a long-handled shoe horn (both from RMS).

Our world is not designed for bigger bodies. I'm talking about too-small chairs or chairs with armrests, booth seats with inadequate space from the table in restaurants, airplane seats, and tiny bathroom stalls, just to name a few. Dealing with these issues is not always in your direct control. The change we must have does not need to be put on you, the individual. If the Centers for Disease Control and Prevention says that 42 percent of Americans are larger in size, why has the world not yet changed to accommodate the needs of this group of people? We need to see change happening at a societal level that accommodates people of all sizes. You wouldn't ask someone in a wheelchair to just fix their legs so they could use the stairs. Instead, you build a ramp to the door.

That said, there are things you can do about these challenges. (1) Practice respecting yourself and standing up for yourself to get your needs met. For example, if you do not want to sit in a restaurant chair that looks too flimsy to hold you or has armrests, ask for a different chair. I know it can feel scary to speak up. Realize that you are not the problem—the chair was not made with you in mind. Bring it to people's attention that you are allowed to take up space too and deserve to have your needs met. (2) Research solutions to potential dilemmas. If you want to travel by plane, find out which airline companies seem to best respect and accommodate fat fliers. Do not let your body size hold you back from living the life you want to live.

For this journaling prompt, focus on the things that you can do to respect your body right now. What are ways you can feel more comfortable in your body at your current size? How do you want to handle future situations that demand you stand up for your needs? Think of an example of when you may need to do this, and write down what you would do or say.

....

....

....

....

MOVEMENT OR REST ACTIVITY

No one is denying the fact that exercise can be great for the body! The distinction here is that you are listening to your body for when exercise is appropriate and creating goals that are not based in weight loss desires. Exercise may or may not change your body size or weight, but it is great for other health reasons. Change your focus to move your body because you enjoy doing it!

For this activity, I want you to make a conscious decision: is today a movement or a rest day? Take account of how your body systems are feeling: Are your muscles sore? Is your digestive system working well? How is your pain level?; and so on. Tune into your body's physical, mental, and emotional energy levels. Do you feel like exercising?

If the answer is no, then today is a rest day. Banish all guilt that comes to the surface with this decision! No matter how many days it has been, honor your body's desire to rest today.

If the answer is yes, determine what movement sounds appealing to you and go for it!

If you are a person who has a strained relationship with exercise (for example, maybe you are someone who never gets the euphoric feeling during/after exercise) but you would like to begin, start with five minutes. If you don't like it, stop. No guilt. Try something else for five minutes the next time you decide it is a movement day. Experiment with all kinds of movement until you find something you like! You don't have to break a sweat or get your heart rate to a certain number of beats per minute. Just notice how your body feels when you try different activities.

Here are a few ideas to get you started:

- Go for a walk (snap some pictures of interesting things along the way).

- Join a pick-up basketball or volleyball game.

- Get some friends together for a game of badminton or pickleball.

- Work in the garden.

- Deep clean around the house.

- Set up an interesting obstacle course.

- Search for YouTube videos that interest you. Be aware that many exercise videos can be triggering or fatphobic. Try finding videos that are demonstrated by someone who has your body type and do not promote weight loss.

- Set up a punching bag for some kickboxing.

- Try yoga or tai chi.

- Rent a paddleboard or kayak and head to the nearest lake.

- Ride a bike.

- Go for a swim.

- Start a foot race with your kids.

- Visit the zoo, aquarium, or local museum for an interesting walk.

- Go to a local farm to pick apples, berries, or pumpkins when they are in season.

- Go skiing, snowboarding, or snowshoeing.

- Find an in-person exercise class. Again be cautious about classes that might trigger or stigmatize you.

- Take your dog to the dog park or for a hike.

Note: If you have a history of over-exercising, I encourage you to skip this activity for now and get your therapist or dietitian's approval before you start any formal exercise.

Prompt

The act of setting a boundary is easier said than done. You have been practicing setting boundaries with yourself while going through this workbook, maybe unconsciously! For example, by agreeing to reject diet culture and stop weight loss attempts, you have set the boundary of not participating in dieting. You have also set a boundary to stop negative self-talk or body shaming.

But your inner voice is not the only thing that will need boundaries. You still live in a world heavily influenced by diet culture and will encounter situations or people that don't align with your new anti-diet views. In time your resilience to diet culture will strengthen, but in the beginning it can be easy to fall back into its many traps. Think of people in your life who are still immersed in diet culture. Maybe they gossip about how much weight so-and-so has gained recently, talk about what new diet looks interesting, or make comments on your body or health. If you are done with these conversations, say so. To set a boundary, you must know what you want and be able to communicate that to the other person.

Remember April's story in Chapter 4 and how her father made remarks about her body and what she chose to eat? April had the self-respect to set the "You don't get to talk about my body" boundary. If you are comfortable doing so, you may choose to educate a person in your life about what you have learned from this book and share your own experiences. Boundaries are hard to set for several reasons: (1) We must acknowledge that our feelings are being hurt because of the actions of others, often loved ones. (2) We may fear what the other person will think of us when we set a boundary. (3) We may fear that the boundary will not be respected. (4) If it is not, we have to decide how to proceed with that person.

You cannot make someone respect a boundary—but there are things you can do. You could start by reminding the person of the boundary you set. After you remind them of your boundary, warn the person you will be distancing yourself from them if they continue to cross your boundary. If that doesn't stop the offensive behavior, then it might be time to detach yourself from the situation: leave the room, hang up the phone (politely if possible), or decline future invitations to spend time with the person. Make sure you follow through on your word.

Broken boundaries can cause big emotions to surface. You have every right to feel disrespected and unheard when this happens. But try not to react or argue with someone who is pushing back against your desire to set or follow through with a boundary. I've found that people who have a narcissistic personality have a harder time respecting boundaries because they hear your words—but they don't care. The best thing to do when dealing with a narcissist is deprive them of attention and distance yourself. You have every right to set a boundary and are allowed to remove yourself from people who make you feel gloomy or triggered.

Are you surrounding yourself with people who bring you positivity or negativity? Who are the people you need to set a boundary with? What boundaries need to be set? Write out a draft of how you will set your boundaries. What will you do if they do not respect your boundaries? What do you need to remember when you are having trouble sticking to your boundaries?

Prompt

Weight stigma is pervasive in health care. Doctors hold the number one spot with women and the number two spot with men as the provider who exhibits the most weight stigma. As scary as a doctor visit can be, you deserve adequate medical care and treatment. In order to make your experience at the doctor's office less anxiety producing, get to know your rights as a patient. Let's break down the most important ones:

1. You have the right to refuse being weighed.

You do *not* have to step on a scale for any reason. Of course, no one is allowed to physically push you onto a scale, but a staff member might be verbally persuasive. I've heard stories of patients feeling forced to get on the scale because the staff claimed a weight was needed for the visit's insurance coverage. This is false. If a staff member claims to need to enter something under the weight section of your chart, tell them to put "refused."

The other option is to close your eyes or step onto the scale backward to avoid seeing the number if it would be triggering for you. Make sure the staff and doctor know that you do not want to know your weight or whether the scale has gone up or down.

There are some medical situations for which a weight actually is required, such as with dosing medication, checking for fluid accumulation (for example, for patients with kidney, liver, or heart failure), or assessing malnutrition. The practitioner can record the number without revealing it to you.

2. You have the right to request that your weight or BMI not be discussed during your visit.

This is a boundary that often needs to be set. If you do not wish for your doctor to discuss your weight or BMI with you, then be frank at the beginning of the appointment. You can say something to the effect of, *Dr. Smith, I would like to discuss my diabetes control today without discussing my weight. I am not actively trying to lose weight at this time, and I would appreciate your opinions on treatment options that are not centered on weight loss.* If your doctor crosses this boundary and still tries to discuss your weight, then you can remind him or her of your wishes. You can also state that you will be looking for a new provider who does not exhibit weight stigma. If you are comfortable, you could also try to educate your doctor or point them to the Health at Every Size and intuitive eating research.

3. You have the right to request a different health care provider.

You have every right to change providers. You can research HAES providers in your area at https://haescommunity.com/search/, check out provider reviews online, and then call your insurance company for a list of in-network providers. Your doctor should be working for *you* and meeting *your* standards, especially because you are the one paying for the visit. You could also call a doctor's office, let them know that you are potentially interested in becoming a patient, but would like the doctor to sign an agreement that they will not recommend weight loss as a treatment option.

4. You have the right to request a copy of your medical records.

Every provider is obligated to provide you with a copy of your medical records. Sometimes there is a fee if the record is large. You can take these records to your new provider if they would find this helpful.

5. You have the right to talk to the clinic manager or other higher-ups within a company.

Unless your doctor owns the practice, he or she is likely not the manager, which means you can voice complaints or point out abuse to someone who may be able to create change. For instance, if your doctor is fat shaming you or refuses to run tests because he or she thinks you just need to lose weight, you can make a fuss. You are likely *not* the only patient getting this kind of treatment. Sharing your experience could have a profound impact on preventing mistreatment of other patients. Make people aware of what is going on behind closed doors.

6. You have the right to leave an online review about a company or provider.

Assuming the company is set up to do so, you can leave a review of your experience on their website or on third-party websites, such as Yelp or Google. There are even review sites created specifically to rate the level of weight-inclusivity of a company. Leaving a review, whether good or bad, will help others looking for the same service. Examples of issues you could address in your review: Were the chairs comfortable and the appropriate size? Were the doorways and hallways comfortable to walk through? Did the staff treat you with respect and dignity? Was the staff friendly? Did you feel heard when expressing your medical concerns? Did your doctor seem informed about the medical issues you discussed? Did your doctor collaborate with you in coming up with a treatment plan? Did you feel you spent an appropriate amount of time with your doctor? Do you feel all your questions were answered and that you understand the treatment plan?

To help make your next doctor appointment feel less scary, write a draft of what you will say or do the next time you are faced with the "weight talk." Decide what you will say to your health care practitioner if they ask to discuss your weight or BMI, recommend a diet for weight loss, or refuse to run tests because of your size. How will setting these boundaries help you meet your needs?

Prompt

You have been learning that there are many ways to respect your body (and yourself). You do this by adequately nourishing yourself, talking to yourself as you would a friend, ensuring physical comfort to the best of your ability, working on your mental and emotional health, setting boundaries, and standing up for yourself to get your needs met.

What does treating yourself with respect look like for you and your body? How are you showing respect for your body today?

FIND WHERE YOU BELONG ACTIVITY

For your last activity, I want you to immerse yourself in a community that supports Health at Every Size and intuitive eating. It could be as simple as following and interacting with fat-positive people on Instagram or Facebook. Or you can search for an offline group of people to surround yourself with. There are Health at Every Size groups all around—or you can start your own. Work to find the support and positive messages you need to stay out of diet culture once and for all. Although you might start out as the one needing the nurturing, you might soon be the nurturer. By sharing your story and experiences, you can help bring others into a place of healing too.

Bibliography

Argilés, Josep M., Nefertiti Campos, José M. Lopez-Pedrosa, Ricardo Rueda, and Leocadio Rodríguez-Mañas. "Skeletal Muscle Regulates Metabolism via Interorgan Crosstalk: Roles in Health and Disease." *Journal of Post-acute and Long-Term Care Medicine* 17, no. 9 (2016): 789–96. https://doi.org/10.1016/j.jamda.2016.04.019.

Bacon, Linda, and Lucy Aphramor. "Weight Science: Evaluating the Evidence for a Paradigm Shift." *Nutrition Journal* 10, no. 9 (2011): https://doi.org/10.1186/1475-2891-10-9.

Berg, Jeremy M., John L. Tymoczko, and Lubert Stryer. "Food Intake and Starvation Induce Metabolic Changes." In *Biochemistry*, 5th ed. New York: W. H. Freeman and Company, 2002.

Cadena-Schlam, Leslie, and Gemma López-Guimerà. "Intuitive Eating: An Emerging Approach to Eating Behavior." *Nutrición Hospitalaria* 31, no. 3 (2014): 995–1002. https://doi.org/10.3305/nh.2015.31.3.7980.

Campos, Paul, Abigail Saguy, Paul Ernsberger, Eric Oliver, and Glenn Gaesser. "The Epidemiology of Overweight and Obesity: Public Health Crisis or Moral Panic?" *International Journal of Epidemiology* 35, no. 1 (2006): 55–60. https://doi.org/10.1093/ije/dyi254.

Choi, Kyung Mook. "Sarcopenia and Sarcopenic Obesity." *The Korean Journal of Internal Medicine* 31, no. 6 (2016): 1054–60. https://doi.org/10.3904/kjim.2016.193.

Cole, Renee E., Heidi L. Clark, Jeffery Heileson, Jordan DeMay, and Martha A. Smith. "Normal Weight Status in Military Service Members Was Associated with Intuitive Eating Characteristic." *Military Medicine* 181, no. 6 (2016): 589–95. https://doi.org/10.7205/MILMED-D-15-00250.

Crawford, D., R. W. Jeffery, and S. A. French. "Can Anyone Successfully Control Their Weight? Findings of a Three Year Community-Based Study of Men and Women." *International Journal of Obesity* 24 (2000): 1107–10. https://doi.org/10.1038/sj.ijo.0801374.

Cruz-Jentoft, Alfonso J., Gülistan Bahat, Jürgen Bauer, Yves Boirie, Oliver Bruyère, Tommy Cederholdm, Cyrus Cooper et al. "Sarcopenia: Revised European Consensus on Definition and Diagnosis." *Age and Ageing* 48, no. 1 (2019): 16–31. https://doi.org/10.1093/ageing/afy169.

Devlin, Keith. "Top 10 Reasons Why the BMI Is Bogus." *NPR*. Last modified July 4, 2009. https://www.npr.org/templates/story/story.php?storyId=106268439.

Dulloo, A. G., J. Jacquet, and J-P Montani. "Pathways from Weight Fluctuations to Metabolic Diseases: Focus on Maladaptive Thermogenesis During Catch-Up Fat." *International Journal of Obesity*, no. 26 (2002): S46–57. https://doi.org/10.1038/sj.ijo.0802127.

"Eating Disorder Statistics." *National Eating Disorders Association*. Accessed July 6, 2021. https://www.nationaleatingdisorders.org/toolkit/parent-toolkit/statistics.

Feldes, Alison, Judith Charlton, Caroline Rudisill, Peter Littlejohns, A. Toby Prevost, and Martin C. Gulliford. "Probability of an Obese Person Attaining Normal Body Weight: Cohort Study Using Electronic Health Records." *American Journal of Public Health* 105, no. 9 (2015): e54–59. https://doi.org/10.2105/AJPH.2015.302773.

Flegal, Katherine M., Brian K. Kit, Heather Orpana, and Barry I. Graubard. "Association of All-Cause Mortality with Overweight and Obesity Using Standard Body Mass Index Categories: A Systematic Review and Meta-analysis." *The Journal of the American Medical Association* 309, no. 1 (2013): 72–82. https://doi.org/10.1001/jama.2012.113905.

Foster, Gary D., Thomas A. Wadden, Angela P. Makris, Duncan Davidson, Rebecca Swain Sanderson, David B. Allison, and Amy Kessler. "Primary Care Physicians' Attitudes About Obesity and Its Treatment." *Obesity Research* 11, no. 10 (2012): 1168–77. https://doi.org/10.1038/oby.2003.161.

Frantz, David J., Craig Munroe, Stephen A. McClave, and Robert Martindale. "Current Perception of Nutrition Education in U.S. Medical Schools." *Current Gastroenterology Reports* 13 (2011) 376–79. https://doi.org/10.1007/s11894-011-0202-z.

Gaesser, Glenn A. "Thinness and Weight Loss: Beneficial or Detrimental to Longevity?" *Medicine and Science in Sports and Exercise* 31, no. 8 (1999): 1118–28. https://doi.org/10.1097/00005768-199908000-00007.

Galloway, Amy T., Claire V. Farrow, and Denise M. Martz. "Retrospective Reports of Child Feeding Practices, Current Eating Behaviors, and BMI in College Students." *Obesity* 18, no. 7 (2012): 1330–35. https://doi.org/10.1038/oby.2009.393.

"Getting Insurance Approval: Arguments to Support Your Claim." *National Eating Disorders Association*. Accessed July 6, 2021. https://www.nationaleatingdisorders.org/getting-insurance-approval-arguments-support-your-claim.

Inoue-Choi, Maki, Timothy S. McNeel, Patricia Hartge, Neil E. Caporaso, Barry I. Graubard, and Neal D. Freedman. "Non-daily Cigarette Smokers: Mortality Risks in the United States."

American Journal of Preventive Medicine 56, no. 1 (2019): 27–37. https://doi.org/10.1016/j
.amepre.2018.06.025.

Jacquet, Philippe, Yves Schultz, Jean-Pierre Montani, and Abdul Dulloo. "How Dieting Might
Make Some Fatter: Modeling Weight Cycling Toward Obesity from a Perspective of Body
Composition Autoregulation." *International Journal of Obesity*, no. 44 (2020): 1243–53. https://
doi.org/10.1038/s41366-020-0547-1.

Jaul, E., Barron, J., Rosenzweig, J. P., & Menczel, J. "An Overview of Co-morbidities and the
Development of Pressure Ulcers among Older Adults." *BMC Geriatrics*, 18, no. 1 (2018). https://
doi.org/10.1186/s12877-018-0997-7.

Kalm, Leah M., and Richard D. Semba. "They Starved So That Others Be Better Fed:
Remembering Ancel Keys and the Minnesota Experiment." *The Journal of Nutrition* 135, no. 6
(2005): 1347–52. https://doi.org/10.1093/jn/135.6.1347.

Keesey, Richard E., and Matt D. Hirvonen. "Body Weight Set-Points: Determination and
Adjustment." *Journal of Nutrition* 127, no. 9 (1997): 1875S–83S. https://doi.org/10.1093
/jn/127.9.1875S.

Keirns, N. G., and M. A. W. Hawkins. "Intuitive Eating, Objective Weight Status and Physical
Indicators of Health." *Obesity Science and Practice* 5, no. 5 (2019): 408–15. https://doi
.org/10.1002/osp4.359.

Lee, Jennifer A., and Cat J. Pause. "Stigma in Practice: Barriers to Health for Fat Women."
Frontiers in Psychology 7 (2016): 2063. https://doi.org/10.3389/fpsyg.2016.02063.

Lupoli, Roberta, Erminia Lembo, Gennaro Saldalamacchia, Claudia Kesia Avola, Luigi Angrisani,
and Brunella Capaldo. "Bariatric Surgery and Long-Term Nutritional Issues." *World Journal of
Diabetes* 8, no. 11 (2017): 464–74. doi:10.4239/wjd.v8.i11.464.

Madden, Clara E. L., Sook Ling Leong, Andrew Gray, and Caroline C. Horwath. "Eating in
Response to Hunger and Satiety Signals Is Related to BMI in a Nationwide Sample of 1601 Mid-
age New Zealand Women." *Public Health Nutrition* 15, no. 12 (2012): 2272–79. https://doi
.org/10.1017/S1368980012000882.

McCleary-Gaddy, Asia T., Carol T. Miller, Kristie W. Grover, James J. Hodge, and Brenda Major.
"Weight Stigma and Hypothalamic–Pituitary–Adrenocortical Axis Reactivity in Individuals Who
Are Overweight." *Annals of Behavioral Medicine* 53, no .4 (2019): 392–98. https://doi
.org/10.1093/abm/kay042.

McIntosh, James. "What to Know About Ketosis." *Medical News Today*. January 24, 2020.
https://www.medicalnewstoday.com/articles/180858.

Montani, J-P, Y. Schutz, and A. G. Dulloo. "Dieting and Weight Cycling as Risk Factors for Cardiometabolic Diseases: Who Is Really at Risk?" *Obesity Reviews* 16, no.1 (2015): 7–18. https://doi.org/10.1111/obr.12251.

Moy, Jordan, Trent A. Petrie, Sally Dockendorff, Christy Greenleaf, and Scott Martin. "Dieting, Exercise, and Intuitive Eating Among Early Adolescents." *Eating Behaviors* 14, no. 4 (2013): 529–32. https://doi.org/10.1016/j.eatbeh.2013.06.014.

Nelke, C., R. Dziewas, J. Minnerup, S.G. Meuth, and T. Ruck. "Skeletal Muscle as Potential Central Link between Sarcopenia and Immune Senescence." *EBioMedicine*, 49 (2019): 381–388. https://doi.org/10.1016/j.ebiom.2019.10.034.

O'Hara, Lily, and Jane Taylor. "What's Wrong with the 'War on Obesity'? A Narrative Review of the Weight-Centered Health Paradigm and Development of the 3C Framework to Build Critical Competency for a Paradigm Shift." *Sage Open* 8, no. 2 (2018). https://doi .org/10.1177/2158244018772888.

Pearl, R. L., and R. M. Puhl. "Weight Bias Internalization and Health: A Systematic Review." *Obesity Reviews* 19, no. 8 (2018): 1141–63. https://doi.org/10.1111/obr.12701.

Pelley, John W. "Nutrition," chapter 19. In *Elsevier's Integrated Review Biochemistry*, 2nd ed. (2012): 171–79. https://doi.org/10.1016/B978-0-323-07446-9.00019-2.

Phelan, S. M., D. J. Burgess, M. W. Yeazel, W. L. Hellerstedt, J. M. Griffin, and M. van Ryn. "Impact of Weight Bias and Stigma on Quality of Care and Outcomes for Patients with Obesity." *Obesity Reviews* 16, no. 4 (2015): 319–26. https://doi.org/10.1111/obr.12266.

"Phentermine." *LiverTox: Clinical and Research Information on Drug-Induced Liver Injury*. Bethesda, MD: National Institute of Diabetes and Digestive and Kidney Diseases (Last updated June 4, 2020). https://www.ncbi.nlm.nih.gov/books/NBK547916/.

Puhl, Rebecca M., and Kelly D. Brownell. "Confronting and Coping with Weight Stigma: An Investigation of Overweight and Obese Adults." *Obesity* 14, no. 10 (2012): 1802–15. https://doi .org/10.1038/oby.2006.208.

Seifarth, C., B. Schehler, and H. J. Schneider. "Effectiveness of Metformin on Weight Loss in Non-diabetic Individuals with Obesity." *Experimental and Clinical Endocrinology and Diabetes* 121, no. 1 (2012): 27–31. https://doi.org/10.1055/s-0032-1327734.

Smith T., and Steven R. Hawks. "Intuitive Eating, Diet Composition, and the Meaning of Food in Healthy Weight Promotion." *American Journal of Health Education* 37, no. 3 (2006): 130–36. https://doi.org/10.1080/19325037.2006.10598892.

Sousa, A., Guerra, R., Fonseca, I. et al. "Sarcopenia and Length of Hospital Stay." *European Journal of Clinical Nutrition* 70 (2016): 595–601. https://doi.org/10.1038/ejcn.2015.207.

Squires, Sally. "About Your BMI (Body Mass Index)." *Washington Post.* June 4, 1998.

"Table: Academy of Nutrition and Dietetics (Academy)/American Society for Parenteral and Enteral Nutrition (ASPEN) Clinical Characteristics That the Clinician Can Obtain and Document to Support a Diagnosis of Malnutrition." *Journal of the Academy of Nutrition and Dietetics* 112, no. 5 (2012): 734–35. https://www.andeal.org/vault/2440/web/files/ONC/Table_Clinical%20Characteristics%20to%20Document%20Malnutrition-White%20JV%20et%20al%202012.pdf.

Tam, Charmaine S., Leanne M. Redman, Frank Greenway, Karl A. LeBlanc, Mark G. Haussmann, and Eric Ravussin. "Energy Metabolic Adaptation and Cardiometabolic Improvements One Year After Gastric Bypass, Sleeve Gastrectomy, and Gastric Band." *The Journal of Clinical Endocrinology and Metabolism* 101, no. 1 (2016): 10. https://doi.org/10.1210/jc.2016-1814.

Tomiyama, Janet A., Deborah Carr, Ellen M. Granberg, Brenda Major, Eric Robinson, Angelina R. Sutin, and Alexandra Brewis. "How and Why Weight Stigma Drives the Obesity 'Epidemic' and Harms Health." *BMC Medicine* 16, no. 123 (2018). https://doi.org/10.1186/s12916-018-1116-5.

Tribole, Evelyn, and Elyse Resch. *Intuitive Eating: A Revolutionary Anti-Diet Approach.* 4th ed. New York: St. Martin's Press, 2020.

Tylka, Tracy L., Rachel A. Annunziato, Deb Burgard, Sigrún Daníelsdóttir, Ellen Shuman, Chad Davis, and Rachel M. Calogero. "The Weight-Inclusive Versus Weight-Normative Approach to Health: Evaluating the Evidence for Prioritizing Well-Being over Weight Loss." *Journal of Obesity* (2014). https://doi.org/10.1155/2014/983495.

Tylka, Tracy L., Julie C. Lumeng, and Ihuoma U. Eneli. "Maternal Intuitive Eating as a Moderator of the Association Between Concern About Child Weight and Restrictive Child Feeding." *Appetite* 95 (2015): 158–65. https://doi.org/10.1016/j.appet.2015.06.023.

Ulian, Mariana Dimitrov, Ana Jéssica Pinto, Priscila de Morais Sato, Fabiana B. Benatti, Lopes de Campos-Ferraz, Desire Coelho, Odilon J. Roble et al. "Effects of a New Intervention Based on the Health at Every Size Approach for the Management of Obesity: The 'Health and Wellness in Obesity' Study." *Public Library of Science One* 13, no. 7 (2018). https://doi.org/10.1371/journal.pone.0198401.

Appendix A

If you enjoyed this book, check out these other amazing titles:

Anti-diet: Reclaim Your Time, Money, Well-Being, and Happiness Through Intuitive Eating by Christy Harrison, MPH, RD. New York: Little Brown Spark, 2019.

Body of Truth: How Science, History, and Culture Drive Our Obsession with Weight and What We Can Do About It by Harriet Brown. Boston, MA: Da Capo Lifelong, 2016.

Body Respect: What Conventional Health Books Get Wrong, Leave Out, and Just Plain Fail to Understand About Weight by Linda Bacon, PhD, and Lucy Aphramor, PhD, RDN. Dallas, TX: Bella Books, 2014.

*The F*ck It Diet: Eating Should Be Easy* by Caroline Dooner. New York City, NY: HQ, 2019.

Health at Every Size: The Surprising Truth About Your Weight by Lindo (formerly Linda) Bacon, PhD. Dallas, TX: Bella Books, 2010.

Intuitive Eating: A Revolutionary Anti-Diet Approach. 4th ed. By Evelyn Tribole, MS, RDN, CEDRD-S, and Elyse Resch, MS, RDN, CEDRD-S, FAND. Ashland, OR: Blackstone Publishing, 2020.

Intuitive Eating for Every Day: 365 Daily Practices and Inspirations to Rediscover the Pleasures of Eating by Evelyn Tribole, MS, RDN, CEDRD-S. San Francisco, CA: Chronicle Prism, 2021.

The Intuitive Eating Workbook: Ten Principles for Nourishing a Healthy Relationship with Food by Evelyn Tribole, MS, RDN, CEDRD-S, and Elyse Resch, MS, RDN, CEDRD-S, FAND. Sydney, Australia: ReadHowYouWant, 2017.

Just Eat It: A Step-by-Step Guide to Escaping Diets and Finding Food Freedom by Laura Thompson, PhD. London, UK: Pan Macmillan, 2019.

Thrive at Any Weight: Eating to Nourish Body, Soul, and Self-Esteem by Nancy Ellis-Ordway. Santa Barbara, CA: ABC-CLIO, Incorporated, 2019.

Train Happy: An Intuitive Exercise Plan for Every Body by Tally Rye. New York: Rizzoli, 2020.

Appendix B
Interview with
Amanda Kieser, LMHCA

Too many people go without proper care because they don't believe they need it or fear the unknown. I wanted to give you, the reader, a glimpse into the world of eating disorders and their treatment. I interviewed a compassionate therapist who works in this field. Amanda Kieser is a licensed mental health counselor associate (LMHCA), who recently finished graduate school and has been working at the Bellevue, WA, Center for Discovery, a residential eating disorder treatment center. As many as six patients at a time reside at the center. This controlled setting and supervision help patients break the cycle of eating disorder behaviors.

(Content warning: Weight-stigmatizing language and numbers are used in this interview.)

Q: What is the primary role of the therapist in treating eating disorders?

A: My role is really to help the person process how the eating disorder has served them or how it has been helpful. A lot of the work is trauma related, and it is not uncommon for coping to become maladaptive over time. I acknowledge that their eating disorder has been a way to cope with a lot of the hard stuff, but show them that it is no longer effective and no longer sustainable. I hold space for my patients who are accepting that and working through it. Patients are often grieving the loss of their eating disorder, and I help my patients sift out what is too tough to manage without their eating disorder. We tease out depression, trauma, and/or anxiety symptoms and help them find new ways of coping.

Q: What types of body sizes do you see?

A: It's a wide range of body diversity for all types of diagnoses.

Q: What does a typical day look like for the patient?

A: They are on a fairly tight schedule that can range from about 5:00 a.m. to 11:00 p.m.; wake-up times are different depending on how many patients are currently there. In the mornings, breakfast is at 7:00 a.m. Then they may have group work or be in session with the therapist or dietitian throughout the day. Some may have scheduled snacks between meals. Free time is in pretty short supply, as there is a lot of work to get through in such a short period of time.

Q: How do you see diet culture and the idea that "thin is best" come across in your patients?

A: Diet culture affects us all and is ingrained in our society and culture's messaging. Even if we think we are not on a diet, or just not affected by it, we really are. There are so many subtle things. Often I talk with my patients about the way social media affects their eating disorder. Everything tells us we have to look a certain way: tall, thin, white, blonde. Diet culture makes us compare ourselves to others and always feel dissatisfied with our bodies and looks. Social media wants you to portray yourself as "always doing well" and doesn't share what is going on behind the scenes. You are never going to be good enough for diet culture.

Diet culture makes it okay to comment on people's bodies and appearance. You are praised for losing weight and looking "healthy." I have to help patients reprogram their brains and question, *Is that okay? Do I need that validation? Is it really anyone's right to comment on how I look?*

Q: Can you describe the ways you have seen the aftermath of patient harm done by doctors or other medical professionals who promote weight loss?

A: Early on in someone's life there can be messaging from doctors who tell parents their child is "obese" or at risk of becoming so. Parents are pushed to fix this "problem." In older clients, we find they are nervous about seeing their health care provider and are anxious or worried that their medical concerns won't be heard. I have one client who lives in a larger body who is scared to bring up her eating disorder with her doctor because in her mind she still believes she needs to lose weight. The dietitian and I have had multiple conversations with her, trying to determine why she still thinks that. Maybe it is a desire to look a certain way. But she feels that the need to lose weight has been reinforced everywhere over her lifetime.

Part of our initial assessment is asking clients if they take any substance or medication to offset appetite. We had a client last year who had been prescribed weight loss medications. She weighed between 140 and 150 pounds at that point. At one point she even sought out getting bariatric surgery. She was very deep in her eating disorder.

We have conversations with the patients, talking about how a medical provider is not the "end-all, be-all authority," and if they are not open to other conversations [besides weight loss] or taking a look at other reasons for their medical problem, it is likely time to switch providers. Or encourage them to do some education around HAES with the doctor if the patient is comfortable with that. Luckily, we have a medical team that we contract with that is knowledgeable in HAES.

Q: What verbiage do you use with someone to get them to see that their behaviors around food and body are dangerous?

A: Diet culture doesn't typically allow us to talk about how awful it feels to be on a diet, so [in treatment] we talk about it. We typically think we are supposed to feel good or at least feel better when we are trying to lose weight or diet. We talk about how dieting behaviors are normal in society and that it may look like people are happy and getting healthy on the outside. But if it's not working for you, it's probably also not working for them. It brings some relief, like, *Oh, I don't have to feel awful about myself that I don't feel great or am not losing weight on a diet.*

We also talk about HAES and that health is determined by a lot of different things. The idea that health is only about weight or BMI is outdated. We talk about if the patient is hiding their behaviors. ED [Eating disorder] behaviors are different from diets in that the behaviors become shameful and often are done in private to keep hidden. I ask patients, "When people are talking about the diet they are on, do you feel like you can talk about your behaviors? Can you tell them you count every calorie consumed? Or that you actually don't eat?" We have to be critical about the things we see and are interacting with. They clearly affect us.

Q: What are some common reasons why people have developed eating disorders?

A: I've commonly seen clients, by virtue of trying to find community, discover others who were struggling with the same issues, such as body dysmorphia—and were trying to change their bodies with restrictive eating or other disordered eating behaviors—and start copying them. Another typical situation is a parent or medical professional sending the message to a child that there is something wrong with them, that they must change their body. It puts fear and fatphobia into the child that translates into an ED later. EDs can stem from bullying or teasing about weight by loved ones or friends growing up. And many times, EDs come out of trauma. It's not uncommon for most of our folks to also carry a PTSD diagnosis. EDs are one way of gaining control and power in one's life. It's also dependable, meaning, *If I do X, I will feel Y.*

Q: Do you find that patients have a hard time accepting a Health at Every Size approach?

A: There is a lot of fear around gaining weight. Clients can be good at holding contradictions; they love the idea of HAES and think that it is great for everybody, but they can't imagine themselves living in a larger body or being at a bigger size. Conversations then quickly become answering the questions of what is it about the fears of gaining weight. There is this distorted thought that if she gains weight, she's going to immediately go from one extreme to the other. Some clients have no insight into how much weight they are actually gaining or losing. If I had to guess, I would say on average, clients gain maybe 10 pounds while they are at the treatment center. But they are thinking they have gained 50 pounds. And that's because body changes are becoming more apparent, and they have to sit with the feeling of being full after eating instead of having a way to release it [through purging].

Q: Can you share a testimony in which inpatient treatment helped a patient on their path to ED recovery?

A: I had one client who had lived in a larger body most of her life and was also very tall. She had this feeling of being too big and taking up too much space. We taught her about mindful and intuitive eating. At first, she really struggled with it because it was difficult for her to detect her hunger and fullness cues after years of inadequately nourishing her body. By the end, she really accepted HAES and her mindset changed to one of believing she was allowed to take up space and allowed to even own the room if she wants!

Another client had weight cycled most of her life. At an early age, she was sent to fat camp and put on diets by her parents. She would lose a lot of weight and be highly praised and reinforced. But with weight regain, the opposite. I would say it was a pretty abusive family environment. Finally, after years of this weight cycling, she came to us because she had just stopped eating regularly. She was twenty-three at the time. We gave her a lot of HAES education and challenged all that reinforcement to look a certain way. We talked about clothing sizes a lot and how it's okay to be a different size, a larger size, between different stores. Toward the end of our time together, we actually got to go on a shopping trip to find clothes that she could purchase for her body, which she was now taking care of, and to help her feel good about the clothes she was wearing. She was really anxious about trying on clothes because she had no idea what size she was at that point. Her goal was to find one pair of jeans, but she walked out of the store with two pairs of jeans, a shirt, and a sweater! She really turned a corner then and grasped onto HAES. The size on the tag was the size of that specific pair of jeans, nothing more!

Q: What advice do you have for someone who is just learning about intuitive eating?

A: Just trust the process. Trust that your body knows when it's hungry, your body knows when it's full. We are taught to deny or postpone those feelings. We are taught it is wrong to feel hungry two hours later after eating. Intuitive eating accounts for the fact that your body is different from any other body on the planet. Trust that your body knows how to keep you alive. Trust that it's okay to be hungry or full, and do not compare yourself to someone else.

Q: Any closing thoughts?

A: Change starts with all of us. Educating others doesn't have to be rude. Point out things when you see them and make a suggestion. I noticed the chair at the chiropractor's office had armrests and a small seat that, for someone like me in a larger body, is uncomfortable to sit in. My chiropractor probably never thought something like a chair could make a difference in someone's care. We can normalize these conversations and cancel our subscription to diet culture. That will be so liberating for our world! Weight bias affects everyone, even people in smaller bodies. Disordered eating behaviors get missed because [a person's] weight is in the "normal" range and they are deemed healthy.

Acknowledgments

To my husband Kurt: Thank you for always believing in my dreams. You are usually the first to hear them and have always supported me no matter what. I appreciate your gentle guidance when I'm at a crossroad, and how you keep me sane on the long and emotional days. I know as long as I have you, everything will turn out okay. Thank you for your unfailing love.

To my sweet Danny: You unknowingly show me every day what it looks like to be a true intuitive eater. Diet culture does not yet influence your eating habits or the way you think about bodies. No matter my size, you love me unconditionally, and I strive to view myself the same way. I love you my boy.

To my parents: Thank you for your listening ears and encouragement. I think fondly of all the discussions we've had over dinner and late into the evenings. You've always supported and showed pride in my endeavors, and I will forever appreciate this.

To my sisters and brother: I couldn't ask for better friends than you. You are there for me no matter what, always encouraging me and inspiring new ideas. Thank you!

To Grandma Marilyn: I wouldn't be where I am today without you! My career choice, business adventures, and even this book are a result of our time spent together at those cooking classes. Thank you for always showing interest in what I do and encouraging me—you and Grandpa Mike both.

To my dear friend and colleague Nancy: You and I became fast friends three years ago. I've always been able to come to you with my ideas, worries, and successes. I am constantly in awe of your wise advice. You are the older sister I never had, and I thank God for you. xo

To my dear friend and colleague Frances: You've always been there to talk through ideas and give me a different perspective on the situation. I think you and I fuel each other's fire for helping people. I'm so grateful to have you in my life, both personally and professionally.

To my editor Ashten: I was so surprised at how fast you picked up my idea for this book. It felt like I blinked and all of a sudden I had a publishing contract in front of me. Your interest in this book truly inspired me and gave me the confidence I needed to get my thoughts onto the pages. Thank you from the bottom of my heart!

About the Author

Brandy Minks received her master's degree in nutrition and dietetics from Washington State University in 2016. She is a Registered Dietitian Nutritionist currently located in Washington state. In her private practice, Brandy helps people break the dieting cycle and find peace with food. She uses the intuitive eating principles, mindfulness, and body awareness to transition her clients to a healthier and happier lifestyle. She is a board-certified nutrition support clinician who provides medical nutrition therapy to clients of all ages and backgrounds from a weight-inclusive perspective. Brandy is a strong advocate for eliminating weight bias in the medical field and proudly works as an anti-diet dietitian for a small hospital. In her free time, Brandy enjoys writing a blog for her website; gardening; playing with her dog, Daisy, and son, Danny, in the yard; and getting together with family. You can follow Brandy on TikTok @brandyminks, Instagram @brandyminks_rd, or Facebook @brandyminksrd.